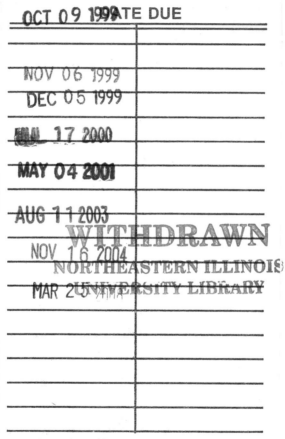

THE ABUSED CHILD

The Abused Child

Psychodynamic Understanding and Treatment

Toni Vaughn Heineman

Foreword by Alicia F. Lieberman

THE GUILFORD PRESS
New York   London

Library of Congress Cataloging-in-Publication Data

Heineman, Toni Vaughn.
    The abused child: psychodynamic understanding and treatment /
Toni Vaughn Heineman.
        p.   cm.   4/8/99
    Includes bibliographical references and index.
    ISBN 1-57230-375-1
    1. Abused children—Mental health. 2. Psychodynamic psychotherapy
for children. I. Title.
RJ507.A29H45 1998
618.92′858223—dc21   98-15497
                                                                          CIP

*This volume is dedicated to Joseph Afterman,
whose career as an analyst, teacher, supervisor,
and consultant has enriched the lives of hundreds
of children and those who care for them.*

Foreword

The treatment of abused children is among the most painful and difficult challenges faced by the clinician. Outrage at the betrayal perpetrated on someone who is by definition in need of protection is inextricably linked with a profound but inherently untenable wish to heal and rescue, to provide the child with a new world where hurts are manageable and adults can help. For the clinician, the emotional burden of recognizing and managing these sometimes overwhelming reactions serves as the backdrop for the more concrete, moment-to-moment struggle of entering into the unique inner world of the abused child, a child for whom trust has been shattered, terror and anger are often uncontainable, symbols can be unrecognizable, and words are insufficient to carry the full force of the experience. The abused child and the clinician at work must move through an internal and interpersonal landscape with few markers, where traditionally sustaining theoretical concepts such as impulse and defense, empathic attunement, transference and countertransference can seem strangely irrelevant and where perpetrator and victim can trade psychological places in an instant, leaving even seasoned therapists in confusion about how to choose and maintain a stance that promotes integration and growth.

Dr. Toni Vaughn Heineman has given us a remarkable "guide for the perplexed" as we make our way in this largely uncharted domain. Her book is an essential resource for coming to grips with the psychic impact of child abuse and for developing ways of working in depth with traumatized individuals of all ages. Her approach transcends theoretical boundaries in its integration of a sound developmental perspective with current knowledge about the neuropsychological effects of trauma, relevant psychodynamic conceptualization, and attachment theory. Dr. Heineman also discusses how to work collaboratively with the parents of an abused child and how to negotiate the often conflicting pressures brought to bear on the clinician by the need to respond to the legal and child protective services dimensions of a case.

But much more than conceptual breadth is exemplified here. Through richly detailed, often brilliant clinical illustrations, Dr. Heineman reminds us that the capacity to tolerate contradiction and ambiguity is among the surest signs of wisdom. She examines, clearly and unflinchingly, the paradoxes that abound in the realm of child abuse—among them, the widespread belief that children don't lie along with the recognition that they can be coached, misunderstood, or misconstrued—and the simultaneous importance of knowing what happened to the child and of moving beyond an emphasis on facts toward an understanding of how the child interprets those facts. The words of Thomas Mann come to mind as we reflect on these mutually enriching yet puzzling polarities: "A great truth is one the opposite of which is another great truth."

The book offers a careful and much needed delineation of the clinical pitfalls confronting the therapist. The twin dangers of premature interpretation and of mistaking a child's ability to describe the abuse with her capacity to connect emotionality to the experience are clearly elaborated through clinical examples. The riches of this book are many, but perhaps its single most important contribution is the thoughtful, persistent, persuasive message that external reality needs to be tethered to an understanding of the child's perception of that reality for authentic, meaning-making inner change to take place. This is a book worth not only reading, but consulting again and again when we need to restore a sense of balance and direction to our work.

ALICIA F. LIEBERMAN, PhD
Professor of Psychology
University of California, San Francisco
Director, Child Trauma Research Project
San Francisco General Hospital

Preface

For over 20 years I have been involved with psychoanalytic theories, as a student, clinician, teacher, supervisor, and consultant. The ideas in this book have evolved over those years. Some of the concepts that I first encountered as a student have remained relatively unchanged in the ways that I think about and work with patients. Other ideas have been set aside when they no longer proved useful. Still other concepts have gone through many transformations through exposure to new ideas I have encountered through reading and discussion. Of course, our ideas—old and new—have little value unless they enhance our clinical work. I am very grateful to the children and adults who, directly or indirectly, in their search for help, have assisted me in trying to separate those concepts that are merely interesting from those that are truly valuable.

I have been extremely fortunate to have had exceptionally talented teachers, students, and colleagues whose eagerness to explore psychoanalytic theory and technique has profoundly influenced my thinking. Acknowledging all of those who have helped and supported me over the years would require several pages. However, I have consistently enjoyed and benefited from spirited discussions with my colleagues Marian Birch, Victor Bonfilio, Diane Ehrensaft, Mary Margaret McClure, Stephen Seligman, and Myra Wise.

I am most especially indebted to Joseph Afterman, to whom this volume is dedicated. His commitment to making the world a better place for children is reflected in the numerous and varied projects he has supported as a clinician and consultant. With thoughtful analytic attention, he has provided guidance in day-care settings and special education classrooms—to parents, teachers, beginning therapists, and advanced analytic candidates. I feel most fortunate to have enjoyed his company over the course of many years, during which he has offered himself as advisor, colleague, and friend with kindness, patience, humor, and respect. To all who know him, he has exemplified the vitality that emerges from continually working to integrate new ideas into theoretical foundations that have stood the test of time and experience.

I have enjoyed the encouragement, help, and support of many people in the process of writing and revising this volume. For careful readings of individual chapters, I thank Daphne de Marneffe, Carina Grandison, and Maria Pease. Eric Stein not only read with care but listened and contributed to this material as it evolved from an idea to a book. The detailed, thoughtful insights of Marian Birch, Richard Ruth, and Bronson West helped me transform the final draft into a finished manuscript. My thanks to my editor, Kitty Moore, who had the confidence to undertake this project when it was little more than an idea on scraps of paper. With unfailing optimism, she shepherded me through the processes of writing for publication.

I also thank my family for their loving support and patience. My children, Parker and Jonas, continually reminded me, as only one's children can, of the value of not taking myself or my ideas too seriously. My husband Alan's confidence in me and this project held when mine failed. His integrity, intellectual rigor, wit, and devotion to the power and beauty of language were most evident in the countless hours he spent editing the manuscript. I thank him for this and for all he has done to sustain me in performing, reflecting upon, and writing about my work.

Contents

They cry in the dark, so you can't see their tears
They hide in the light, so you can't see their fear
They give & forget, all the while
    love & pain become one & the same
    in the eyes of a wounded child

—PAT BENATAR, "Hell Is for Children"

Introduction

In the pages that follow I explore, from a number of perspectives, two seemingly contradictory positions regarding the psychodynamic treatment of abused children: First, aspects of the therapy of abused children will differ in either kind or degree from our work with children who have not been traumatized by abuse. Second, we have no need of special formulas exclusively for physically, sexually, or emotionally abused children. I believe that both of these statements are true. It is the tension between them, our attempts to hold both simultaneously, and our efforts to integrate both these positions into our work that enable us to be most effective as we try to help children to overcome the consequences of abuse.

Regardless of the origins of a child's emotional distress, as therapists, we offer ourselves to children as people who can address their psychological pain. In this way, we approach abused children as we would any other child who comes to us for psychotherapy; simultaneously, we recognize that because the origins and consequences of physical, sexual, and emotional abuse extend far beyond the psyche, our understanding of the child's distress will also have to extend beyond the psychological. The acts that produce an abused child's emotional distress vary enormously, as do the individual children's reactions. Sometimes the abuse has stopped before the child comes to us; sometimes it is not discovered until the therapeutic relationship is solidly established. At times the abuse is grotesquely and obviously brutal; at other times, it is so subtle and insidious that we cannot detect it, let alone stop it. Even when the abuse is eliminated from the child's life, either by actual physical removal from the abusive environment or by significant change in the perpetrator's behavior, the child's suffering continues. The depth of children's pain and the extent of its symptomatic manifestations often surprise and overwhelm even psychologically sophisticated adults. Like the children who come to us for help, we often wish and behave as if both the suffering and its symptoms will pass quickly.

Unfortunately, our desire to minimize the consequences of abuse finds little support from research or clinical practice. The torment of abused children, even with treatment, is not easily attenuated. Over and over again, research in the fields of neurobiology, endocrinology, cognition, developmental psychology, and trauma, as well as psychotherapy research and practice, has demonstrated the forceful and lasting effects of abuse on young children. Their psychological and physiological processes become destabilized in extraordinary ways as a result of abuse. The creation of new, stable states of equilibrium does not come easily to these children nor to the caretakers, teachers, or therapists trying to help them reorder and organize their lives. This is not to suggest that we cannot or should not attempt to alleviate the symptoms that plague abused children as quickly as possible. However, we must view an early abatement of symptoms cautiously, lest we confuse symptom and problem.

We simply cannot learn the fullness of feelings and ideas that follow from abuse in the matter of a few weeks or in a few sessions spread over several months. Nor can we erase the consequences of abuse by informing children about their innocence or teaching them how to avoid "bad touch" in the future. If we do assume that effective treatment of abused children can come quickly or easily, we will certainly not succeed. Furthermore, by colluding in a doomed process, we also unwittingly reinforce the belief, virtually universally held by abused children, that their defectiveness is beyond repair.

However, if we can offer children the time and space to show and tell us who they are and how they came to be, we can help them find ways to correct the damage they suffered at the hands of another. Only by allowing the traumatic influences to unfold in the context of the therapeutic relationship can therapist and child together begin to examine the child's perspective on the abuse, its embodiment in his psychic life, and his struggles to keep it at bay. Psychoanalysis and psychoanalytic psychotherapy emphasize listening and talking, recognizing the need to make meaning of even the most irrational feelings and behavior. In their attention to the complexities of affective relationships, these treatment modalities are uniquely effective in helping children understand the nature and particular meaning of the abuse they have suffered. And then, as they can integrate these events into the multitude of experiences that form the fabric of each individual history, they can begin to move beyond the effects of abuse.

Because there is no single psychoanalytic theory, treating a child who has been abused, from a psychoanalytically informed perspective can and does take many forms. From its inception, the psychoanalytic community has been involved in spirited debates about the universe of emotions, the nature of individual psychology and its relationship to universals within the human psyche, the workings of conscious and unconscious processes, the influence of intrapsychic processes and interpersonal relationships on development, the establishment and maintenance of a sense of self, the creation of mental health and illness, and the means by which those suffering emotional distress can be helped to overcome their difficulties, to name but some of the important issues that excite psychoanalytic discussions.

Differing schools of thought have made an abundance of ideas and techniques available to clinicians. These choices simply would not be possible within a unified psychological theory; at the same time, the sometimes contradictory richness can also overwhelm the unwary student or therapist. The ideas and clinical vignettes in the pages that follow show influences of drive theory, ego psychology, attachment theory, developmental theory, object relations theory, and trauma theory, though not in equal measure. In one vignette, the importance of the child's attempts to ward off overwhelming anxiety by a variety of unconscious strategies or defenses might be prominent, while in another, the emphasis might be on the character of the child's internal world of self and others, the nature of the child's object relationships, or the effects of trauma on neurological processes. These presentations of clinical material, along with the discussions of theory and technique, are intended to demonstrate the ways in which one can select among varieties of psychoanalytic theories and integrate them into clinical work. This is not designed to be a textbook on psychoanalytic psychotherapy with abused children; it is intended to offer a variety of perspectives that can be brought to bear on understanding and treating children who have been physically, sexually, or emotionally violated.

Private meanings and understandings of child abuse always arise from the particular experiences of the individual. However, they are also embedded in historical and cultural views of children and sexuality, as well as in economically and politically determined attitudes toward victims and those who harm them. The first three chapters provide the theoretical foundations for the later discussions of psychoanalytic treatment of children and the particulars of working with children who have suffered abuse.

Chapter 1 offers a delineation of the relationship between abuse and psychological trauma. I also provide a brief consideration of differing historical and cultural attitudes toward the treatment and maltreatment of children.

In Chapters 2 and 3, I sketch an overview of psychoanalytic perspectives on child development, including self-representations, the child's object relationships, and patterns of cognitive growth. Using clinical examples, I argue the crucial importance of situating any diagnosis or treatment of an abused child in a developmental context.

Although neurological processes form the substrata of private meaning making, they do not always receive adequate attention in the consideration of symptom formation and cure. Chapter 3 presents the basic elements of neuroanatomy and neurobiology that seem especially influenced by traumatic abuse. This background allows us to examine the physiological elements of some of the symptoms, such as affective disregulation, flashbacks, and impairments in memory and learning, commonly associated with abuse.

In Chapters 5, 6, 7, and 8, I identify some facets of treatment that differ from therapy with other child patients and that matter deeply enough to warrant special consideration. The core of the therapy may well lie in how the child remembers (or not), defends against (or not) and verbalizes (or not) her experiences of being abused.

Thus, in Chapter 5, I reflect on the memories, or lack thereof, of abused children, or of adults who later report having been abused as children. These often raise perplexing questions for clinicians as well as for the legal system. I discuss some aspects of children's memories and their relationship to the instability of fact and fantasy as discrete categories in children's lives. This leads to a consideration of why some children disclose abusive incidents while others do not.

Chapter 6 looks at the origins and purposes of dissociation as defense against the painful knowledge of and affects arising from abuse.

Here I also examine externalization as an equally powerful, though less often discussed, force in the lives of abused children.

The relationship of action to spoken language has particular weight in the psychoanalytic treatment of abused children. In Chapter 7, clinical material illustrates variations in children's capacities to narrate aspects of their internal and external lives. Chapter 8 details some of the very confusing, intriguing, difficult, but inevitable, interplay of feelings between therapist and child that arise in clinical work with abused children.

In the final three chapters, 9 through 11, I step back from the immediate work with abused children to consider the impact of abuse on those in the child's environment, especially the people on whom these children are most reliant. Clinical material is used to demonstrate the strength of the influence abused children exert on those around them.

Chapter 9 addresses some of the complications that abuse introduces into the work with parents or substitute caregivers. By focusing on those very painful situations in which, despite our best efforts, we are powerless to change the course of an abusive history, Chapter 10 reemphasizes the critical importance of early and thorough intervention with abused children. Finally, because we are often asked to help the courts evaluate children and families in which there have been allegations of abuse, in Chapter 11, I examine the process of court-ordered evaluations. This chapter elucidates the importance of our creating time and space for the story of child and family to unfold.

Many years ago, when I was a trainee at San Francisco's Mt. Zion Hospital,* I was in a case conference with a senior analyst. During this conference, one of the trainees would typically present clinical material for group discussion. At one particular meeting, the presentation prompted an especially lively and somewhat heated discussion among the beginning therapists who made up the group. Anxious, uncertain, and eager to impress each other and the conference leader, we argued among ourselves for some time about the correctness of a certain

---

*We enjoyed the great benefit of a multidisciplinary training that integrated graduate students at various levels of education and training—interns/residents/fellows—from social work, psychiatry, and psychology into the entire didactic and clinical curriculum.

interpretation. As was his wont, the leader listened quietly but did not contribute to the debate for some time. When our conversation had run its course, he mused, "Whatever happened to just sitting quietly with people and their feelings?"

Today I have no idea what interpretations we considered or whether we ever agreed whether one was better than another, let alone why. But that simple question has come to mind countless times over the ensuing years, particularly in work with those who have suffered abuse, where connections are so terrifying that our words and feelings are turned aside while the explicit and implicit demands for action are often intense. It has helped me to remember to sit quietly when I have nothing to say. It has reminded me that although my words may sometimes fall on deaf ears, I can remain connected to the person I sit with if I am attuned to the feelings in the room. It has also helped me to know that when I don't feel in touch—don't understand the other person or what passes between us—just sitting there may be enough. It has helped settle me when I feel lost in a torrent of actions, words, and feelings.

The abused children who come for help require so much from us. In the following pages, I have tried to demonstrate how, from this position of quiet reflection, we can come to learn all of the story, both spoken and unspoken, that abused children bring to us as well as why, if we attempt to act too quickly—to exercise our skills or demonstrate our knowledge—we fundamentally undermine the therapeutic process. I trust that this volume will assist those who work with abused children by contributing to their knowledge and skills. Most important, I hope it will heighten their appreciation of the value of sitting quietly with another.

Chapter *One*

What Is Abuse and Who Decides?

Unfortunately, children's lives are sometimes beset with accidental or inadvertent trauma. Some traumas result from human error and therefore, at least in theory, might have been avoided. The fatal crash of an automobile or airliner may remind us of the fallibility of our bodies and our machines. A natural disaster that claims dozens or even hundreds of lives may remind us of our mistaken beliefs in the power of human beings to predict or control the forces of nature. Although they may cause physical and emotional trauma, accidents and natural disasters are neither deliberate nor personal. The hurricane or the flood does not intend to hurt those in its path; the drunk driver does not consciously choose his victim.

In contrast, abused children are deliberately chosen and intentionally hurt. Except in the wildest stretches of a child's imagination, abusive behavior cannot be construed as accidental or impersonal. However, in desperate attempts to avoid the knowledge that the abuse was neither impersonal nor accidental, children do stretch their minds to construct explanations beyond all credibility. Even if numbers of children are brutalized by a teacher or if all of the girls in a family function as their father's sexual partner, each specific attack against each individual child is personal and deliberate. Herein lies one of the paradoxes of child abuse: Abused children often justifiably feel as if they have been treated as impersonal objects—merely used for the expression of another's sexual or aggressive impulses. Simultaneously, each child is unique and will experience and internalize the abuse in a profoundly personal way. Because abuse denies the essential "personhood" of the child, this can lead to the incorrect conclusion that the abusive actions were not deliberately inflicted on an individual child, that is, that a child or group of children were harmed largely because they happened to be in the wrong place at the wrong time. While external circumstances may make some children more vulnerable to abuse than others, physical, sexual, or emotional abuse cannot and should not be construed as accidental, as devoid of intent.

Abuse does not occur between equals. The very use of the term suggests an inequality in the balance of power in the relationship. "Child abuse" connotes both the severity of mistreatment and the actual helplessness of the victim in relation to the perpetrator. The fluidity often found in abusive relationships sometimes leads to the erroneous conclusion that children share in the responsibility for the abuse inflicted upon them. Even when there is mutual brutality between parent and child, we cannot hold the child to the same standard of responsibility. Children do not have real power over their parents or other adults. Their power is illusory. It is granted, whether deliberately or unintentionally, by those in actual power. When an adolescent throws hot coffee in her mother's face, the incident may appear to be a fight between equals. When the mother punishes her daughter by beating her with an extension cord, she reasserts her actual power. When a child proclaims that she consented to or even invited sexual contact with an adult, she erroneously disavows her need for actual adult protection while wrongly asserting her mistaken view of herself as capable of mature judgment.

In our attempts to understand the horrific actions that adults can inflict upon children, we sometimes confuse unconscious motivation with lack of intentionality. We may erroneously suggest that if the perpetrator did not knowingly intend to hurt his victim, the actions do not constitute abuse. Unfortunately, abuse *can* and *does* result from the opposition of a stated positive aim and an unconscious ill intent. It is precisely the pairing of stated benign or positive intent with unconscious malevolence that is paradigmatic of child abuse. The mother who feeds her son poison in order to kill the demons within him does not knowingly wish to harm her child. Indeed, her stated purpose is to save him. If we see her behavior as unconsciously motivated by a rage that she cannot allow herself to know, we might feel some sympathy for a mother so tormented by her own impulses and feelings that she must retreat into psychosis. However, regardless of the mother's conscious intention or unconscious motivation, her behavior is abusive.

At its most extreme, abusive behavior demands little consideration of the intentions or motivations of the perpetrator. When cigarette burns cover a child's body, we can be confident that the child has suffered physical abuse; when a child's vagina and rectum show severe bleeding and scarring, we can equally confidently assume that she has suffered sexual abuse (Bays & Chadwick, 1993).

However, these are not the cases that raise questions for clinicians. The stories that make us wonder about the children's internal processing of these assaults to their bodies are those that lie on the edges of the adult–child relationship. At what point does a spanking become a beating? What transforms sexualized play into sexual abuse? How do we differentiate between a "time out" that merely exceeds a child's developmental capacity to tolerate being alone and a "solitary confinement" that constitutes emotional abuse? While some, but not all, physical symptoms of abuse can be measured and quantified, the psychological aspects of mistreatment are more ephemeral and more dependent on subjective experience.

Our clinical judgment must include consideration of the child's subjective experiences, which is not to say that we must mold our opinion to meet the child's. I do not agree with the premise that feeling abused and being abused are identical or interchangeable. Both parents and children easily become confused about the meaning and consequences of their actions. A mother who impulsively swats her 2-year-old as he dashes toward the street may suffer pangs of guilt, feeling that she has been abusive. A 10-year-old may complain bitterly that being deprived of a longed-for activity is unreasonably harsh, even cruel punishment, despite her repeated and apparently deliberate disobedience of her parents' rules. The child whose mother frequently and unpredictably unleashes a tirade of viciously demeaning fury at him may feel that he earned these tongue-lashings, but he does not understand the distinction between deserved punishment and emotional abuse. The little girl whose father gently and sensually caresses her entire body may not feel any reason to complain of mistreatment, particularly if that activity forms the basis of their relationship, but this treatment will have lasting effects even if she doesn't label it sexual abuse.

Judgments about whether specific actions or patterns constitute abuse depend, not only on the particulars of the behavior or the severity of the mistreatment, but on the extent to which the person initiating the action recognizes and respects the child as a separate and dependent entity with distinct needs and desires. In those instances of subtle mistreatment, the action moves into the category of abuse when the perpetrator's behavior privileges his or her needs or desires above those of the child to such an extent that the person with authority denies the separate existence of the child. I concur with Shengold (1989, pp. 1–2) that this, along with feelings of unbearable intensity in response to mistreatment by someone in a position of power are the essential conditions of child abuse.*

A mother who sends a boisterous child to his room because she needs a bit of peace and quiet puts her needs ahead of the child's; this not only does not constitute abuse—it may prevent it! However, the mother who locks the noisy child in a dark closet for several hours is acting entirely for her own benefit; at that moment, her needs make it impossible for her to consider the needs or desires of the child. Thus, in a bizarre and twisted way, although child abuse always involves at least two characters, in the mind of the perpetrator, the child ceases to exist.

Abuse robs children of their humanity; it disavows the very essence of their being in what Shengold (1989) so aptly termed "soul murder." I have yet to encounter, nor can I imagine, a case of child abuse that could, in any way, be understood as benefiting the child. This is not to say that I have not heard and read numerous rationalizations for abusive behavior. In every case, the explanation seems so clearly a futile attempt to render rational the deliberate use of the child to satisfy the needs of the perpetrator. In the most egregious instances, the rationalizations, whether psychotic or merely patently self-serving, are blatantly unbelievable. A mother explains that she beat her child to the point of unconsciousness to teach her not to cry. A minister describes having a young girl fellate him in order to bring

---

*This is a clinical, not a legal definition. There are instances of mistreatment that a clinician might label "abuse" that would not meet the requirements for prosecution.

her closer to God. A father routinely humiliates his son in public to teach him to respect his elders.

When incidents like these distinctly fall outside the bounds of consensually validated norms, we can easily recognize that the abusive behavior had everything to do with the adult's emotional state or needs and nothing to do with the emotional, physical, or social needs of the child. However, abused children are often offered rationalizations such as these. First violated and misused, then told a bizarrely twisted story explaining that their suffering is for their benefit, they are dishonored yet again, sometimes more deeply by the pretense than by the behavior (Carlin et al., 1994; Conte, 1995; Delahunta & Tulsky, 1996; Fenton, 1993; Friedrich, 1993; Heineman, 1994).

When children hear "This is for your own good," they know to expect something disagreeable. When adults tell children that "This hurts me more than it does you," it rarely does. In the face of the lies that frequently accompany abuse, the child must hold her sense of integrity by herself alone. To preserve her essential sense of herself, she must know and bear the ugly truth—that she is being used solely for the needs of the other—by herself. Embracing the lie means surrendering her soul along with her body. However, paradoxically, accepting the lie also offers her a way out of her aloneness—if she agrees, even tacitly, that her abuser recognizes her as a distinct entity whose separate and actual needs are served by the abusive behavior, then there is a "meeting of the minds." This truly awful choice of surrendering psychic integrity and reality in order to preserve relatedness can and does drive children mad.

Insanity is only one among many consequences of child abuse. Depression, anxiety, sexual dysfunction, aggressive behavior, nightmares, insomnia, poor physical health, learning difficulties, and the inability to form or maintain relationships are among the consequences of abuse that plague children long after the actual abuse has stopped (Fergusson & Lynskey, 1997; Beck & van der Kolk, 1987; Halgin & Vivona, 1996; Ashworth, Fargason, & Fountain, 1995; Burland, 1994; Krystal, 1985; McCauley et al., 1997; Miller, McCluskey-Fawcett, & Irving, 1993; Reber, 1996; Summit, 1983; Terr, 1990, 1991). We are only beginning to appreciate the ways in which children carry these harms into adulthood and pass them along to others.

Although most abused children do not become abusive adults,

most abusive parents were, themselves, abused children. This "cycle of abuse" is widely recognized. However, it is less commonly understood that the interpersonal consequences of child abuse are much more wide-ranging. Anyone who has been mistreated by a victim of child abuse has suffered the indirect effects of that person's malevolent past.

The horrors of child abuse usually serve to keep us focused on the child, herself. Perhaps because what she endured has been so great, we feel guilty for giving any attention to those who suffer only indirectly and much less severely. However, when the abused child goes to school and hits his classmates at the least provocation, they too become victims of child abuse. The teacher whose self-esteem declines when that child repeatedly thwarts and ridicules her genuine efforts to reach him also sustains the effects of child abuse. When that child grows up and routinely mistreats coworkers and those who would befriend him, they, too, become indirect victims of child abuse, as do the partners of women who, because of the sexual abuse they suffered as children, cannot fully enjoy the pleasures of sexual intimacy as adults (Finkelhor, Hotaling, Lewis, & Smith, 1989; Moeller, Bachmann, & Moeller, 1993).

This is not to suggest that any sharp word or inconsiderate act arising from a victim of child abuse can or should be attributed to the abusive past; it is to remind us that us that the pain of child abuse cannot be contained within the abused child.

As Karen's behavior vividly illustrates, many innocent bystanders are also hurt by child abuse, some inconsequentially and some more seriously. As clinicians, we are trained to recognize and work with the sources of our patients' pain without succumbing to its harm. However, most of the people in our patients' lives do not know how to protect themselves from the mistreatment that follows in the wake of child abuse. In the presence of someone who has not overcome the consequences of an abusive past, they may quite literally feel as if they "don't know what hit them."

Karen

Karen entered psychotherapy during her freshman year in college because she found herself panicked and unable to concentrate during any school holiday or extended break. She feared that without the structure of school she would go mad. As a month-long winter break loomed on the horizon, her anxiety reached such a pitch that she could not sleep and lived her days in a state of physical and mental agitation. She had refused her internist's offer of medication. She didn't know exactly why, but the thought of "not feeling" frightened her even more than her terrifying feelings.

Karen could not contain her painful desperation. If a man responded to her flirtations and seductive behavior, she often physically attacked him when he moved to kiss or caress her. On other occasions, she mistook an innocent conversation as evidence of a man's romantic interest in her and pursued him, almost to the point of stalking. Karen could not keep friends because of her extreme reactions to any perceived slight; she once threw all of a housemate's belongings out the apartment window when he ate some food that she had put in the refrigerator. When a professor warned her that she was in danger of failing a class if she did not turn in a required paper, Karen became so enraged that the professor, fearing for her own safety, called campus security to have Karen removed from the office.

These people did not understand the terror that prompted Karen's erratic and irrational behavior. They didn't know that even slight triggers could send her swirling into a fragmented world of flashbacks in which she felt as if she were fighting for her life. They protected themselves as best they could—by getting away from her—but not before they had been hurt. Although the physical and emotional injuries Karen inflicted on others did not compare to those she herself had suffered as a child, they hurt, nonetheless.

Karen described growing up in an extremely religious family. The church had formed the center of her family's social life. They spent at least one evening a week and all day Sunday at church. Dancing, card playing, tobacco, and alcohol were prohibited, and young people were strongly encouraged to socialize within the church group. Premarital sex was absolutely forbidden, yet the surprise weddings of adolescent couples occurred frequently in this congregation. More often than not, a baby followed within a few months. The minister who had led the congregation throughout Karen's childhood and adolescence had resigned after confessing to impregnating a 15-year-old girl. Karen recalled that she and her friends all "knew" that this man offered special prayer meetings to some of the adolescent girls in the congregation. She had felt both relieved and rejected when she had not been invited to participate.

She now wondered if the adults, too, had both known and pretended not to know about these meetings as well.

Karen remembered being routinely sexually molested by an older cousin and his friends during most of her childhood and early adolescence. At times she felt very guilty about this, reasoning that if it had gone on for so long, she probably had been at least partially willing to participate in this activity, which she knew to be sinful. Karen's mother confirmed her memory of asking for help in stopping her cousin. She had admonished Karen to stay away from her cousin and his friends, reminding her that "boys will be boys." Later Karen's mother was astonished to learn that the abuse had continued beyond this conversation. She explained to her daughter that because Karen's complaints had stopped, she had assumed that the molestation had stopped as well.

Along with demonstrating the profoundly destructive effects of child abuse, not only on the immediate victims, but on those who later enter their lives, Karen's story also shows the importance of context in understanding the unique meaning of any individual experience of abuse. In some stories of child abuse, figure and ground are relatively stable, and the abuse is an aberration in an otherwise healthy environment. Unfortunately, in Karen's case, as in so many of the stories we hear about child abuse, figure and ground continually fade into each other, making it impossible to separate definitively the consequences of abuse from the effects of the environment in which it occurred.

Karen, like many abused children, did not live in an otherwise healthy environment. Her parents' attention to the family business and church activities left them little time or energy for their children. In addition, the family's social milieu promoted an atmosphere of deceit and hypocrisy. In the church's stated position, all church members were held to equally high standards of behavior; yet the implicit message from both family and church was that men and boys just can't be expected to control their impulses. This left the real responsibility for obedience to the rules to the girls and women. The unspoken but very powerful message was that boy's sexual exploits are understandable, but only "bad" girls, that is, those who want sex, will make themselves available to them. Karen's uncertainties—whether she had wanted to be one of the minister's "special" girls, whether she actually had been molested or whether she had willingly joined in her cousin's activities because she just wanted sex—were certainly under-standable given the confusing and contradictory environment in which she grew up.

Throughout history, all manner of tortures have been inflicted on children for the stated purpose of education, moral edification, increasing their physical or sexual prowess, or correcting their errant behavior (Coppolillo, 1987). At other times and in other cultures, the mistreatment of children stemmed from their lack of value in the marketplace or work force—like animals, their worth depended on their capacity to produce (deMause, 1998). The more distant in time and the more different the modes of mistreatment are from currently accepted norms, the easier it is for us to separate ourselves from those who hurt children (Erdoes & Ortiz, 1984; Hamilton, 1940; Ions, 1983), either purposely or inadvertently, in the name of religion, science, or a philosophy of child rearing. We shudder at the thought of infants being deliberately exposed to the elements in order to toughen them up, children offered as sacrifices to appease the gods, boys being castrated in order to preserve their voices for cathedral choirs, or girls being forced into prostitution to support a family.

However, history does not allow us the comfort of seeing such behavior as aberrant (Breiner, 1990, Meadow 1993a, b; Hicks & Gaughan, 1995; Gillenwater, Quan, & Feldman, 1996). The abuse and mistreatment of children has often enjoyed widespread social sanction. The children who labored to the point of death in Dickens's England were neither the first nor the last to work as virtual slaves so that the more affluent could enjoy the spoils of their labor (Shengold, 1988). While we now have laws to protect against the exploitation of children in our own work force, manufacturers, who go abroad to save on labor costs, may well perpetuate the forced labor of children in third world countries to work excruciatingly long hours in unhealthy conditions.

We may become uncomfortable when learning of ancient cultures that supported brother–sister incest as a means of children exploring sexuality or advocated the manipulation of children's genitals in order to prepare them for sex with adults. However, the socially sanctioned use of children for the sexual pleasure of adults is not comfortably confined to the past. Today, tiny girls are dressed as sexy miniature adults to participate in beauty pageants, and the Internet offers ready access to groups that profess the benefits of indoctrinating young children into the world of sexuality.

Our discomfort over the mistreatment of children is perhaps most painful when we consider the abuses that have risen from our own ranks. While it might now seem woefully harsh and misguided, the practice of confining children in elaborate and painful devices to prevent masturbation, supported by medical and psychological professionals, is not so distant. More recently, mothers of even tiny infants were admonished to feed their infants only every 4 hours and to refrain from offering comfort when their babies cried lest they raise "spoiled" children. Currently, in some quarters, children who have been diagnosed with a severe attachment disorder are subjected to therapy that includes forcing them into physical submission or depriving them of air until they lose consciousness. These techniques stem from an understanding that children carrying this diagnosis have never learned and cannot, except under extreme conditions, learn to trust or rely upon another, that is, to form an attachment. These methods have as their ostensible purpose teaching children to love.

It is easy to identify the flaws in the psychological theories and techniques from other times or other cultures; we are perhaps more likely to overlook or be blind to the conceits and dangers in our most recently embraced approaches to treatment. However, when we face the history of our attitudes toward children, including the prescriptions and remedies that professionals have offered to parents and teachers, as well as our direct treatment of our young patients, we are forced to recognize that children have not always fared well in the hands of adults. Perhaps our most important lesson is to approach our work with humility. The truths that seem so self-evident today may tomorrow appear ineffectual, laughable, or even destructive.

Chapter Two

Developmental Considerations in Evaluation and Treatment

Children grow. This simple, obvious fact sometimes eludes our notice; we may fail to consider what it means, how it affects a child's view of the world, or our view of the child. The extraordinary childhood neurological growth described in Chapter 3 manifests itself only indirectly; we don't see the brain grow and change, but we do observe the consequences of neurological development, both during "critical periods" of rapid growth and times of consolidation, through the behavioral changes that take place from infancy through late childhood.

Physical growth is more easily observed, both by parents, who wonder how clothes can be so quickly outgrown, and by children, who eagerly measure their increasing height against that of friends, siblings, parents, or the chart from last year's trip to the pediatrician. Physical skills change dramatically over the course of childhood. The glee of a child's first tentative steps echoes in his later prowess on the soccer field, basketball court, or dance floor; from the infant's pincer grasp, increasingly refined fine motor control allows for mastery of pen and pencil, the computer keyboard, videogame controls, paintbrush, or guitar strings.

We notice cognitive and language development, too. We marvel as the child travels from naming familiar objects to reading simple sentences to composing complex essays or moving poetry. By the end of elementary school, the child, who once happily counted beans or dolls or marbles without regard to one-to-one correspondence, can perform complex calculations with whole numbers, fractions, decimals, and percentages. An egocentric view of the world gives way, at least most of the time, to an exercise of the logical principles underlying a scientific world view.

From only a rudimentary awareness of an "other," the child gains an understanding of relationships within her immediate and extended family. Divorce, death, and remarriage of parents, siblings, aunts or uncles may force an unwelcome intimacy of knowledge about why and how relationships dissolve as well as how they are sustained. Peer relationships change from a young tot's reliance on playmates available because of proximity, whether at home, day care, or in the neighborhood, to friendships made at school, neighborhood centers, in sports activities, religious groups, community organizations, camps, or clubs. Socially, the child develops the capacity to hold an independent place in a variety of communities, some of her parents' choosing, some of her own making.

By late childhood, children understand and appreciate fair play and can even tolerate "bending the rules" to accommodate less skilled or younger children. Generally, they have learned the rules of the family and society. In examining their behavior, they look not only to their parents or other adults for approval or disapproval but experience a sense of pleasure or displeasure emanating from their own conscience.

The global affective responses of infancy give way to an intuitive understanding of the subtle nuances of emotional interchanges. Emotionally, the child evolves from utter dependence on others for care to a substantial capacity for self-care and independent activity. Of course, even though a child *can* feed the dog, remember her homework, or express anger verbally rather than through a tantrum, it doesn't mean that she always will. And when she does act like an amazingly competent being throughout the day, it does not mean that she will not want a bedtime story or an old, almost forgotten, lullaby that night.

Because children live in this world of rapid developmental transitions and reorganizations, we frequently encounter more difficulty in comprehending their responses than those of adults. The constant state of flux, sometimes greater, sometimes less, in their emotional, social, and cognitive capacities necessarily adds a degree of uncertainty to our psychological understanding of their behavior. In addition, children, more than adults, are vulnerable to regression in the face of both internal and external stresses. Because of the instability of neurological processes in young children, newly acquired skills are particularly vulnerable to disruption in the face of stress. Physiological factors such as illness, lack of sleep, hunger, or abuse as well as psychological factors such as intrapsychic or interpersonal conflicts can cause children to lose developmental ground. We cannot always easily determine whether behavior or mood is a temporary consequence of developmental shifts, a transitory response to an external event, or a more serious symptom of developmental and psychological disruption.

Perplexed teachers and parents often come to us precisely because they are uncertain about how to interpret the meaning of a child's behavior. Two-year-old Johnny starts spanking and shouting at the toy animals at the day care center. Does this mean he's been spanked at home? If he has, does it mean he's been physically abused? Dana, who is 4, wants Jimmy to play doctor, which involves a complete physical exam, without clothes. Is this indicative of sexual overstimulation? Five-year-old Tom cries every time his father picks him up at kindergarten. He complains fearfully that his father is mean, that he "hates" going to his father's house and only wants to stay with his mother. Is Tom's father doing something he shouldn't be doing?

Psychodynamic theories (Tyson & Tyson, 1990; Ainsworth, Blehar, Waters, & Wall, 1978; Cath, Gurwitt, & Ross, 1982; Chodorow, 1978; Erikson, 1950, 1980; Freud, 1963, 1965; Mitchell, 1991; Seligman & Shanok, 1996, Winnicott, 1971) of child development provide the foundation from which we can begin to answer these and the many more complex questions parents, teachers, and children present to us. An awareness of the predictable sequential stages of human development allows us to appreciate the symptomatic deviations that follow child abuse. Neither a single beating nor a single sexually abusive act are isolated intrapsychic incidents; they continue to influence the course of the child's development. Abused children suffer the effects of mistreatment for many, many years and in complex ways.

Abuse occurs in the evolving representational history of the child; neither the child's psyche, nor its neurological substrate, are static environments. Once introduced into the child's internal world, abuse, like other influences both beneficial and noxious, becomes an internal part of the child's psychic life. The abusive experience is constantly being reevoked, reworked, and reformulated in relation to the changing interdependent landscapes of the child's mind, neurobiological reorganizations, and information emanating from the external world. At times the influence of abuse on the child's behavior, thoughts, dreams and daydreams will be quite evident, while at other periods, its effects may rest more quietly in the background of the child's psychic life.

Thus, while we must approach abused children as victims of noxious *external* events, the internal experience of abuse is ultimately created by the child. This is not to suggest that abuse is somehow only what children make it to be but that any child's experience of abuse will be unique, both in the manner in which it is first absorbed and understood and in the ways it is psychically "metabolized" over the course of development.

When we demand consideration of a child's developmental status in trying to understand the effect abusive experiences might have on her, we are merely reminding ourselves that the resources available to a child who must endure and try to come to terms with abusive experiences will vary over time. Since true emotional and cognitive growth inevitably brings changing views of historical and psychic reality, it makes sense that abuse, whether a single event or a painfully chronic aspect of childhood, will be reconsidered, both consciously and unconsciously over the course of development. Indeed, history is rewritten retrospectively, sometimes many times over. For example, a child whipped for soiling when she is 3, may attribute the whipping to her having "messed" herself. Later, when her sexual curiosity blossoms, she may remember or reinterpret that very same incident as due to her "messing with" herself.

Abusive incidents, like other externally generated events, are always received by the child not only through the emotional and cognitive tools available to her at the moment but through the developmental lens that dominates at the time. As clinicians, we are obligated to try to grasp the reality of the abusive events and the meaning the child made and continues to make of them.

For example, when sisters, ages 2 and 7, are repeatedly told to behave themselves at dinner, then are spanked when their continued horseplay results in a pitcher of spilled milk, their internal responses to the spanking, considered solely from a developmental perspective, are likely to be very different. When their angry father announces that the spanking was punishment for disobedience and carelessness, the two children's fantasies about the "true" crime that induced the angry smacks will be highly influenced by the developmental issues of the moment. The 2-year-old, struggling to master her aggressive feelings and impulsive behavior, may associate the spanking with her father's anger earlier in the meal when she stubbornly pleaded that she was big enough to pour her own milk. Her older sister, who developmentally is more likely to be striving for a sense of cognitive and social competence, may respond with a sense of humiliation over both acting and being treated "like a baby." Since her developing conscience is probably still relatively harsh, she may berate herself for this mishap or silently blame her little sister for getting her into trouble. Later in the evening, if the pull is toward identifying with the punitive parent, she might feel quite justified in beating up her little sister for some real or imagined misbehavior. If she is drawn toward an identification with the helplessness and innocence of children, she might, given an opportunity, offer solicitous comfort to her younger sister. Abusive experiences gain their extraordinary psychological power from the confluence of physiological responses and developmentally generated meanings.

From the inception of a psychodynamic theory of development, clinicians and researchers alike have worked to refine our understanding of the course of childhood and to integrate observations and research from different disciplines into psychoanalytic perspectives on intrapsychic processes. Like human development, psychoanalytic developmental theory is in a continual state of flux, invigorated by new experiences and information. Over time, new data render some concepts useless, while others draw strength from ongoing research and clinical material. In the knowledge that behavior and the neurological processes underlying it cannot be isolated except for semantic purposes, I have taken the liberty of focusing on the relatively predictable emotional and behavioral changes that characterize child development in this chapter and of examining neurological development in Chapter 4.

The available literature on human development fills volume upon volume; it would be both pointless and impossible to summarize our current understanding in just a few pages. However, I believe it is important at least to touch on some of the salient aspects of the different developmental stages from infancy through the early elementary school years. Rather than providing an academic approach to this topic, for example by considering physical or cognitive factors in each phase, I have tried to highlight the issues and behavior that best characterize each stage, using clinical material for illustration. I offer these rudimentary descriptions of emotional development both as a backdrop for considering the impact of abuse at different periods and to suggest that a developmental perspective provides a language for addressing children as we try to help them integrate abusive experiences into their unique developmental journeys.

INFANCY

Spending even a short bit of time with an infant makes clear why infancy is sometimes termed the "oral phase." Indeed, in addition to the pleasure gained sucking at the breast or bottle, infants explore the world with their mouths; their own fists and thumbs go into their mouths, as do the noses and fingers attached to those holding and playing with them. Along with the pacifiers or teething toys they accept from solicitous parents or siblings, babies also happily mouth the slimy bone left behind by the family dog, an older brother's toy, or grandfather's glasses case.

For physical as well as emotional survival, the infant depends not only on the nutrients gained from sucking but on the tactile and visual stimulation intrinsic to affectionate interactions during feeding. From birth, the human infant is uniquely adapted to enter into increasingly complex patterns of reciprocity and mutual attachment with her parents. (Schore, 1994; Stern, 1985; Greenspan, 1988). For example, the infant's greatest visual acuity sits at the approximate distance between her and her mother's face while nursing. Thus, in a "good enough" relationship, the infant's intense oral pleasure becomes intertwined with the comforting, pleasurable image of her mother. Looking, then, also becomes pleasurable as mother and infant repeatedly engage in mutual gazing, gaze aversion, and reengagement. These intensely pleasurable affective experiences, in turn, enhance the development of the visual cortex.

Because of his immature nervous system, the newborn infant responds to bodily sensations and external stimuli in relatively disorganized and holistic ways. With extremely limited capacities for consciously deliberate and discrete communication, the young infant depends almost entirely on the ability of parents or other caretakers to recognize and minister to his needs. When parents do correctly assess and meet a child's needs, feeding him when he is hungry, changing him when he is wet, or comforting him when he is distressed, mutually determined patterns of interaction gradually evolve between parent and child. The importance of reciprocity in the increasingly subtle and sophisticated lines of interdependent communication on an infant's behavioral and neurological organization cannot be overestimated.

While the greater burden of establishing reliable patterns of communication obviously falls on the adult who is in dyadic relationship to the infant, both controlled studies and careful observations of parent–child interactions have increasingly taught us that the infant also plays a crucial role in establishing relationships (Beebe & Lachman, 1992; Greenspan, 1981; Call, 1964; Brazelton, Koslowski, & Main, 1974; Stern, 1985). For optimal development, not only will the baby have a "good enough mother" (Winnicott, 1958), but the mother will have a "good enough baby." For example, premature infants, whose signals are less differentiated and predictable than full-term infants run a greater likelihood of being the target of physical abuse (Frodi et. al., 1978). A parent–child dyad comprising an easy-to-read baby, an attuned parent, and a comfortable temperamental fit will have much easier time establishing a mutually satisfying, reciprocal relationship than will a parent–child dyad in which any one of these factors is less favorable.

For example, those infants who quickly develop differentiated cries and establish behavioral patterns make it relatively easy for parents to read their cues and respond appropriately. The parents then receive reinforcement from the infant and develop a sense of competence and confidence. As parents' confidence in their ability to assess and meet their child's needs increases, they are more able to tolerate the frustrating times when they cannot easily read or soothe their baby. In turn, the infant comes to associate the sight, sound, and smell of his parent with the cessation of discomfort and the initiation of soothing comfort. In this way, the parent–infant dyad creates reliable neurological processes for affect regulation.

When a baby's cries are disorganized or relatively indistinguishable or when she is not easily soothed, it places her parents in the frustrating and upsetting position of trying to guess which of many possible needs or wishes she is trying to communicate by her wails. If they offer food and she continues to cry, perhaps she is not hungry, but perhaps her response to satiation is delayed. Because this baby's cues do not always clearly indicate her needs, her parents must rely heavily on their own judgments and intuitions until they can more readily anticipate the baby's signals. If parents often must try a number of strategies to soothe their unhappy baby, never quite sure what their child needs, they will find predictable interactions difficult to estab-lish. In turn, the baby will take longer to associate different bodily states with responses from the environment. For example, until she learns that food relieves one, but not all, internal discomforts, she will have trouble distinguishing hunger from other unpleasant internal states. Fortunately, most parent–infant pairs adapt to each others rhythms and temperaments more or less easily and with enough success to create a backdrop for the infant's healthy development.

However, for some dyads, what each contributes and needs from the relational interactions differs so dramatically that successful adap-tation becomes exceptionally difficult. Some babies are easily over-stimulated and quickly distressed when their environment is not relatively peaceful. Suppose this kind of infant has a mother who is innately talkative, active, and quick to respond to any sign of upset. Her instinctive approaches to her infant may contain more stimulation than he can manage, leading to a cry or other expression of upset, which in turn activates his mother's futile attempts to minister to him. When her attempts to soothe him fail, she may well become increas-ingly discouraged, distressed, or even lose emotional and physical control.

Unfortunately, adults who were abused as children may be more likely to find themselves ensnared in this kind of unsatisfying, frustrating, and potentially dangerous parent–child relationship. One of the long-lasting neurological consequences of abuse (see Chapter 4) is difficulty in regulating affective responses. Even when this symptom has been greatly ameliorated, pathological responses can be reevoked in affectively charged situations. It is not difficult to see how a vulnerable parent could be moved to a state of hyperarousal, prepared for quick, life-preserving action by a baby's cries. As we know, the parent in that state of physiological arousal does not make a very good judge of the real dangers posed by the immediate environment. So when the parent experiences an intensification of anxiety, even to the point of panic, she may feel mounting pressure to take ever stronger actions in order stop the baby's cries and her own rising discomfort.

Moreover, the psychological residue of abuse may cause the parent to interpret the cries as evidence of a "bad baby" and to use this as justification for punishing the wailing child. Thus, in some cases, we might see an abused parent's mistreatment of an infant not only as a desperate attempt to stop the physical and emotional distress she herself is experiencing in response to her crying infant but also as a bizarre, but psychologically determined, effort to maintain or restore a positive image of her own abusive parent. If her baby deserves punishment, then she, like her own parent, will be acting quite reasonably in disciplining the child's intentional misbehavior (Newberger & Cook, 1983; Newberger & deVos, 1988). In other instances, a parent who has been abused may identify the baby with her own abusive parent and, experiencing the baby as abusive (Benedek, 1959), attempt to avoid the crying child or punish the infant as she could not retaliate against her parent.

In addition to relating to their infant as an individual with distinct physical and personality traits, parents also assign children various roles depending on differing identifications. These may be conscious as, for example, when a child is described as having "her grandmother's eyes" or being "just as stubborn as his uncle." Sometimes these identifications are relatively fixed and impervious to change in the face of external reality. As a result, a little boy might be described as "stubborn" even when he is not, or he may meet his parents' expectations and actually become an obstinate child. Many adults who were abused children come to parenthood with an unstable sense of self and a fluid matrix of internalized relationships and identifications. In these cases, the infant can, in the parent's mind, quickly move from good to bad, from self to other, from grateful to demanding. Like *The Ghosts in the Nursery* described by Fraiberg, Adelson, and Shapiro (1975), the following case demonstrates the dangers that can befall a child when the roles the parent has assigned to him are both malevolent and unconscious.

Deborah and Sam

Deborah gave birth to her only child, Sam, at the age of 19. As a child, Deborah had suffered through frequent stays in boarding schools and foster homes, beginning at the age of 3. During intermittent periods of living with her parents, her father frequently crawled into bed with her and softly stroked her legs and genitals; she remembered feeling his erect penis against her as he sang her lullabies. Following her father's death, her mother remarried and had a second child, whom both her mother and stepfather favored. During her late childhood Deborah had frequently been slapped and verbally berated by her mother, a successful and well-known artist. By early adolescence Deborah had been actively suicidal; by late adolescence she had left home and married a man many years her senior.

Deborah's responses to her own infant fluctuated between complete indulgence and furious tirades. Throughout much of Sam's infancy she carried him, strapped in a sling next to her body, from dawn till dusk, putting him down only long enough to change him. At night, Sam slept between his parents so that he could nurse whenever he wanted.

Generally, Sam was a happy baby who was quickly soothed. However, like any other infant, he sometimes just cried, despite Deborah's every effort to calm him. She found his wails so unbearable that she would scream that he was "an ungrateful wretch" who should be sent to an orphanage until he learned how lucky he was to have a mother who loved him. When her husband attempted to intervene, either when things were calm, by suggesting that perhaps Sam didn't need to be held every moment, or during one of Deborah's rages, she turned on him. If he suggested that she needn't indulge Sam quite so fully, Deborah excoriated his "accusations" that she was an unfit mother; if he tried to interrupt one of Deborah's verbal assaults on Sam, she attacked him for siding with their "greedy, ungrateful bastard."

By the time Deborah brought Sam for consultation at the age of 3, things had gone from bad to worse. Sam's parents had divorced, but they continued to fight bitterly. Sam continued to nurse on demand. He had been "expelled" from every play group or nursery school Deborah found because of his utter inability to conform to even minimal standards of behavior. The teachers worried about his well-being as well as the safety of the other children. Sam climbed as high as possible on every available structure whether or not the construction was designed for playing. If Sam wanted a toy that another child wouldn't relinquish, he might easily throw a chair across the room or slam his fist in the other child's face. When teachers tried to restrain him physically, he became frantic—hitting, kicking, and shouting that they were trying to kill him.

When Sam didn't get his way with Deborah, he would hit her and run out of the house. He refused to stay in bed when put to sleep, often running around the house until the wee hours of the night, sleeping wherever he collapsed. Deborah's efforts at discipline, which usually began with reasonable expectations and limits, quickly escalated to screams and threats of long-lasting, horrible punishments. Her tirades only escalated Sam's frenzy. At these times Deborah routinely took Sam, kicking and screaming, to his father's, threatening that she wouldn't see him again until he learned some discipline. However, she would usually arrive to pick him up a few hours later, worried that the father's parenting skills were more suited to military training than the raising of young children. Sam's father was a strict and demanding, although not cruel or abusive, man; however, he had little chance to try to exercise control over his anxiety-ridden son.

Over a long course of intensive psychotherapy, Deborah came to recognize that unconsciously she continued to cling to her childhood conviction that she had suffered abuse in response to her inherent badness and unreasonable behavior. Indeed, like Sam, she had been an extremely ill-behaved child, making it easy for her to concur with her mother and stepfather's assertions that she "deserved" the punishment she got. She tried to be the perfect mother for Sam. Sam, of course, inevitably failed to be the perfect infant. She then saw him in the same way that she had viewed herself as an infant and child—as bad, demanding, greedy, and ungrateful. For Deborah, the terrifying alternative was to hold herself responsible for her behavior, and, by extrapolation, to hold her own mother responsible for *her* behavior. The unconscious world of abused children often demands either a bad parent or a bad child. Because the idea of a "bad parent" is entirely untenable, the child will create a good parent, no matter what the actual circumstances. Thus, the only explanation for beatings, verbal humiliation, or unwanted sexual advances, must be that the child "asked for it."

Sam's placement in a day treatment program enabled him to get help in understanding and controlling his own terrifying aggressive impulses. Gradually, he came to relinquish his need for omnipotent control and could accept reasonable limits from his parents and other adults. Fortunately, through individual, family, and milieu therapy, Sam and his parents were able to overcome the very grave effects that his mother's abusive childhood bestowed on his infancy. Even though everyone considered the outcome successful, it was definitely not the beginning one would want for any child.

TODDLERHOOD

The transition to walking as the primary means of locomotion ushers in toddlerhood. As the youngster teeters on the brink of competence in gross motor skills and mastery of the rudiments of spoken language, those around her gradually come to see her as emerging from the world of infancy and beginning the complex physical and emotional naviga-tion of childhood. In this period of separation–individuation, young children show unsurpassed glee in their new-found abilities to propel themselves through space. However, their joy can easily turn to fear or sadness if they are allowed to venture too far, whether physically or emotionally, from the safe haven of parental attention. The increased capacity for locomotion is intimately linked with the fundamental emotional tasks of the toddler—establishing a sense of autonomy while maintaining connections using distal modes and internal repre-sentations despite physical and temporal separateness (Lieberman, 1993; Mahler, 1974; Settlage, 1980). He can move away from and return to his parents; he can hold them in his head and heart when they are physically or emotionally at a distance.

As his gross motor skills develop, the blossoming young child can manage his own affairs increasingly well. He can begin to feed himself and, for example, in addition to making his likes and dislikes known by tossing unwanted food on the floor, can give verbal expression to his dietary preferences. With patience and practice, the toddler learns to dress himself and often expresses firm ideas about what is fashion-able and what is not. Along with preferring the same foods day after day, children of this age often insist on wearing a favorite outfit for days on end, dissolving into tantrums or tears if a parent insists on more "appropriate" or clean attire. It is unfortunate that toddlers have had to live under the rubric of "the terrible twos." Their characteristic feisty stubbornness, viewed less pejoratively, can be seen as crucial in their move toward independence and a stance that maintains the courage of their convictions. Their staying power in the face of reasoning, cajoling, bribery, anger, and threats of punishment can be truly remarkable.

Locomotion allows for the child's physical separation from the parent. Object constancy, the developing capacity to hold a stable image of the parent, in the midst of both positive and negative feelings, permits the toddler's increasing emotional autonomy. If a parent habitually withdraws in the face of a child's insistent "I can do it myself," or routinely and bitterly refuses to comfort a child in the wake of a temper tantrum, it will make it difficult for the child to hold a consistent and reliable image of the parent, and her capacity to separate will be compromised.

Considering what is at stake, we should not be surprised that an exhausted child of 2 or 2½ will vehemently insist that she does not want to go to bed, that she is *not* the least bit sleepy, despite having missed her nap and being up well beyond bedtime. For her increasingly impatient parents, this may seem like a simple matter of adhering to the rules and making sure that child and parents alike get enough rest. From the child's point of view, she is engaged not in an inconsequential debate about bedtime but in a fight for her autonomy, a battle over her claim to her own existence. As she becomes increasingly aware of and in control of her body, she is concomitantly less eager to have others tell her how to manage it! As in the example above, the child may protest particularly strongly when she is tired because the regressive pulls of sleep and the old comforts of infancy arise with special intensity.

Understandably toddlers protest most fiercely against their parents. It is from their parents that they must separate while simultaneously forging a relationship that can accommodate their budding autonomy. Of course, the toddler's recognition of his parent as a separate being accompanies his learning about his own separateness. About the former, he is, at least initially, generally displeased; about the latter, ambivalent. The acceptance of the child's autonomy also causes conflicts for his parents, who must, like the child, relinquish the shared pleasures of infantile narcissism and then join him in the joys of his growing independence.

The toddler's move toward autonomy might be thought of as analogous to a colony's declaring its independence from the motherland. While neighboring countries may simply honor the new country's request for independent status, the previously sovereign state, even if it acknowledges the colony's capacity for self-rule, may be reluctant to relinquish its actual power and the sense that the mother country alone has the experience and wisdom to govern—not to mention the benefits of total devotion and dependence.

Children of 2 and 3 often feel in the grip of a life and death struggle against the very people they love most in the world and from whom they are trying to establish a modicum of independence. Their "adversaries" also feel ambivalent about the outcome of the struggle, both treasuring the child's growing competence and mourning the passing of the warm dependency of infancy. We can therefore readily appreciate the extreme complexity of this conflict, which will require many skirmishes in order to reach a resolution. This ambivalence, which contains aggression within a mutually loving tie, is a hallmark of healthy parent–toddler interactions.

Toddlers reside in what Freud (1905/1953) aptly called the "anal phase" because of the physical pleasures associated with bowel and bladder functions. Toilet training naturally constitutes one of the primary interactional tasks navigated by toddlers and their parents; though it offers the opportunity for both parties to feel a sense of triumph, the process may also lead to anger and frustration. Toileting is among the first demands parents place on a child for self-care and involves their suggesting where and when he should deposit his bodily products. Meanwhile, the child is developing a sense that he should be in charge. Consequently, we would be quite surprised if these interactions didn't produce some parent–child disagreements. Indeed, the struggles over control form an important and inevitable part of toddlerhood, even though they may drive even the most patient parent to distraction.

In my experience, if a parent who does not believe in spanking is going to be reduced to hitting a child, it is most likely to occur during the later phase of the child's toddlerhood. Unlike the younger toddler, whose babyish manner offers her a measure of protection, the older toddler seems more like a child than an infant. So, while the protests of a 12- or 18-month-old over being dressed or having a diaper changed may frustrate and annoy, his stubbornness lacks the sophistication and willful defiance that a child of 2 or 2½ can bring to a disagreement. Parents of toddlers often complain of feeling diminished or undone by their children's anger and obstinacy. The frequency of comments like, "I can't believe I was reduced to the level of a 2-year-old," indicates how easily parents of toddlers can begin to feel as out of control as their youngsters.

When a parent's childhood struggles over impulse control are ignited by an unruly child, that parent may unconsciously identify with the child and not only feel childish but resort to childish behavior such as yelling, throwing, or hitting. Fortunately for Mickey, his father was able to control his impulses, but his efforts to do so poignantly show how fiercely parents must sometimes fight to maintain discipline themselves in the face of a toddler's provocative behavior.

Mickey and His Father

It is Saturday afternoon, and Mickey's father has taken his son, approaching his third birthday, to the playground. They spend about an hour playing together, but his father allows Mickey to pick the activities. Mickey clearly enjoys his father's help, attention, and admiration. Though an hour of pushing his son on the swing, catching him at the bottom of the slide, and helping him navigate the junior monkey bars gives the father pleasure, it also eventually bores him.

After a while, the father suggests that he'll sit for a few minutes and read the newspaper he has with him. Mickey pays little apparent attention to his father's announcement and goes on with his play. A few minutes later, he calls for his father to watch him on the slide. The father glances up and waves. Mickey calls for help; his father responds that he should try it himself. Mickey calls again, this time near tears. Realizing that he is not going to get any reading done, the father resigns himself to another, though shorter round of play.

Nap time approaches. After a bit, the father announces that it will soon be time to go home. In anticipation of Mickey's protests over leaving the park, the father is pleased to remember that he has one of Mickey's favorite snacks waiting on the kitchen table at home. When he gives Mickey another warning that they must soon leave, he reminds Mickey that they can have chocolate pudding when they get home. Mickey nods and runs for the swing, calling for his father to push him. The father agrees but stipulates "just one more time." Again with great patience, the father gives a warning, declaring that there will be "ten more pushes." Mickey gleefully joins his father in counting down to "blast off." He obligingly leaps down from the swing and with an anxiously excited laugh runs for the slide, leaving his father to contend with the failure of his patiently constructed strategy to make the leave-taking easy for both of them. The father's tolerance begins to give way to annoyance as he chases after Mickey. When he finally scoops him up in his arms, Mickey's laughter turns to wails of protest. The father's humiliation and helplessness make him acutely aware of other parents watching him, alternately feeling their glances as sympathetic and critical. At this point, he only wants to be at home, with Mickey soundly asleep in his bed.

Despite his best efforts, the father's mood shifts to a silent determination not to be manipulated by the temper tantrums of a 2-year-old! As his rage mounts, he considers increasingly stringent punishments "to teach Mickey a lesson." However, before he has time to act, he recognizes that his thoughts of vengefully reasserting his authority stem in part from feeling that Mickey has taken charge of the outing. He feels aghast at the harshness of the punishments he has imagined to reassert his parental authority. The recollection of the extent of his anger adds guilt to the range of emotions he has encountered in this brief Saturday outing to the playground.

Mostly out of guilt for his anger at his son, the father tries to atone for his "sins" when they arrive home by offering Mickey the pudding. Mickey stubbornly declines the peace offering and is summarily and angrily put into his bed for a nap. After a bit his father recognizes that the sound of Mickey's cries have changed to forlorn tears. He decides to wait a few minutes, then goes to Mickey's room to comfort him and to verbalize how upset both of them had been. The father expresses his own sadness that their trip to the playground, which had been so much fun at the beginning, had ended so badly. He adds that they would both have to work harder on stopping, even when they were having fun, and not getting so angry. When Mickey asks for his snack, his father says that he doesn't really think this is a very good time for it, but that he will get Mickey a glass of water and sit with him for a few minutes. He offers to put the pudding in the refrigerator so they can share a snack after Mickey wakes from his nap. Mickey awakes refreshed to a father who, having had time to rest and compose himself, is again delighted to see his son.

Stories like this strike a familiar chord for those who treat young children or for the parents of toddlers. In this case, Mickey's father was able to contain both Mickey's rage and his own, even in the face of Mickey's deteriorating loss of impulse control. However, Mickey's father felt pushed almost to his limit; when relaying the story to his counselor, he confessed that, had he not been walking down a street in his own neighborhood, he probably would have "smacked" his son. Fortunately, he didn't; even more fortunately, he expressed interest in examining the motivation for his wish to do so.

When parents describe, whether sheepishly or proudly, responding to a child's hitting, biting, or kicking with similar behavior, they are often unconsciously trying to "get even" with the child for making them feel small, childish, and helpless. These reactions may be justified with rationalizations like, "I just wanted to give him a dose of his own medicine," or "Maybe if he knows how it feels, he'll think before he bites somebody else."

Suggestions that inflicting physical pain may not be a viable means of discipline seldom serve much purpose. Therapists who attempt an educational approach to this situation often find themselves engaged in a power struggle with an entrenched parent, who holds to her argument with all the ferocity of a willful 2-year-old. Because the argument that she was acting in a reasonable way is unconsciously designed to protect her against the feelings of helpless rage engendered by her child's behavior, she cannot accept the childishness of her behavior without first acknowledging the childishness of her feelings. If the therapist becomes increasingly adamant in her insistence on discussing alternative forms of discipline, the power struggle naturally repeats itself, with the parent now taking the role of the obstinate 2-year-old who will not listen to reason and the therapist acting out the role of the long-suffering, increasingly frustrated parent.

Unfortunately, therapists caught in this position will commonly act out their unconscious hostility toward the parent who has successfully passed on to them a feeling of utter helplessness. When we carefully examine these situations, we can often clearly discern that the therapist's behavior mirrors the parent's behavior toward the child. For example, the therapist may unconsciously become extremely inflexible about scheduling appointments, then interpret the parent's protests or absences as a failure to cooperate. If the therapist has not resolved her own conflicts over aggressive impulses, she may unconsciously create an atmosphere in which the parent comes to feel constantly in danger of being cited for child abuse—that her requests for help when she has erred will be reported as abuse or that when she announces that she has *not* hit her child, she will be accused of being in a state of denial and therefore still guilty of abuse.

For parents who were themselves abused as children, raising a toddler leaves them vulnerable to intense feelings about the inherent badness of their own aggressive impulses. They can easily interpret their child's striving for autonomy as no more than willfully defiant attempts to undermine their authority. They may alternately see their children as the abusive parents of their own childhoods, as they themselves were as children, as the personification of their own aggressive impulses, or as a danger to their own weakening controls. Just as they were confused as children about whether their behavior warranted beatings, or scalding hot showers, or hours locked in a dark closet, they may confuse their child's self-assertion with enraged disobedience. Then, rather than consciously identifying with a parent who was abusive or cruel, they see the child as pathologically aggressive. Of course, when they then punish the bad child they felt themselves to be, they have identified with the abusive parent.

THE PRESCHOOL CHILD

Even though the toddler enjoys multiple and varied relationships, his internal world is essentially dyadic; that is, although he sees *himself* in relation to others, he has relatively little interest in the relationships people have with each other. Not until the preschool years does the child's internal world expand into a network of complex relationships. This shift from feeling himself in exclusive relationship to the important people in his life begins with his understanding that his parents each have not only a relationship with him but also a relationship with each other that excludes him. This is a profound psychological discovery, the assimilation of which forms the primary emotional task of the preschool child (Loewald, 1979, 1985; Fonagy et al., 1991; O'Shaughnessy, 1988).

The child cannot fully grasp the nature of a triadic relationship that includes two generations without the cognitive capacity to grasp the concept of past, present, and future. This allows her truly to understand for the first time that her growing up will be concomitant with her parents' growing old. Her earlier egocentricism had allowed for a rather naive view of the world in which she could grow and change while her parents would remain just as she had always known them. In this primitive world view, development occurs in a vacuum that does not alter either intrapsychic or interpersonal relationships.

When this fantasy is lost to him, the young child can feel somewhat bereft as he glimpses himself growing up and moving into the world previously occupied only by parents and other "grown-ups." These cognitive and intrapsychic shifts are paralleled in the child's interpersonal relationships. His expectations of and demands on his

Mary

Four-year-old Mary was referred for evaluation by her preschool teacher, who was concerned that her excessive shyness interfered with the successful development of social relationships. During one of the diagnostic interviews, Mary spontaneously went to the doll-house, where she played quietly for some time. The doll family moved through a rather uneventful day of getting up, going to school, and eating dinner together. Eventually bedtime arrived, and Mary put the mother doll and a little girl doll in bed together. She said calmly that the mother and girl were sleeping together. The child then put one of the male dolls into the bed next to the little girl doll. The child giggled and seemed anxious as she pushed the three dolls together into a writhing mass. The therapist, aware that the mother had a new boyfriend, commented, "Maybe something like that has happened to you." Mary looked startled, left the doll play, and drew listlessly for the remainder of the session. The therapist saw Mary's leaving the dollhouse as a play disruption, evidence that the "disclosure of sexual abuse" was so anxiety provoking that she couldn't continue her play.

Unfortunately the therapist's premature assigning of meaning to Mary's play substantially interfered with the diagnostic process and a clear understanding of the workings and meanings of Mary's intrapsychic processes. While this child may indeed have been playing out something that had occurred in her external life, she may alternatively have been using play to describe her feelings and fantasies about her mother's new boyfriend and what happens in the world of adult sexuality. Perhaps, rather than being joined in the bed by this man, she had been displaced from a bed she had previously shared with her single mother. In this case, the play might have represented her wish to be included in the coziness of the parental relationship rather than endure the solitude to which their relationship had relegated her.

When the therapist made an assumption that Mary's play was a reflection of events in the external world, she either excluded or minimized the possibility that the writhing mass might be a representation of Mary's sexual fantasies and curiosity. The therapist's premature assumption about the meaning of her play seemed to have frightened Mary. This is an understandable response, particularly if a fantasy is incorrectly interpreted as representing reality. Since young children easily move between the two and retain at least a partial belief that some wishes magically come true, an ill-timed or inaccurate interpretation can leave the child with the chilling sense that her fantasy may indeed become real.

Our reasonable concern to attend to even the subtlest clues children offer about abuse or molestation can, with unfortunate consequences, lead us to concretize children's communication. Particularly when confronting the active internal lives of children who, developmentally, are appropriately concerned with sexual themes, it is essential that we respect the importance of fantasy in children's attempts to master concepts and feelings that are difficult for them to assimilate.* Paradoxically, this attempt to take seriously all of what children tell us sometimes results in the assumption, usually unconscious, that children's play and talk reveals only what has happened to them, as opposed to what has happened and continues to happen *within* them. When we too quickly or falsely accept fantasy as standing for external reality, children are understandably confused and frightened. Young children easily move between fantasy and reality, often relying on fantasy to mitigate the unpleasant constraints of reality until those limits can be mastered more effectively. However, when the two fade into an inseparable morass—the beloved parent cannot possibly be searing a cigarette into her child's flesh, but *is*; the man raping a little girl cannot possibly be her father, but *is*—children lose the ease of movement between fantasy and reality. When the worst of a child's fantasy becomes reality, the child can no longer rely on this internal retreat for comfort or a resource for mastery of the inevitable blows of external reality.

LATENCY

The knowledge gained during the preschool or oedipal years offers children a new degree of freedom. As they relinquish the view of themselves as the single most important person in their parents' lives and affections, they gain the freedom to explore new relationships

---

*In this context, it is interesting to note how frequently even adolescents or young adults drolly comment that they know that their heterosexual parents "did it" at least the number of times that correlates with the number of children in the family. Children's appreciation of their parents' pleasure in sexuality comes very slowly indeed.

with both peers and adults. This is essential to the successful psychological move outside the family to the world of school and friends (Sarnoff, 1976).

The sexual curiosity and preoccupation of preschool children are gradually transformed during the early years of elementary school into increasing interest in the world beyond the family. This is not to say that a 7- or 8-year-old child is not intensely involved with and affected by the events and feelings in her home, but rather, that her cognitive capacities, physical skills, and increasing reliability in autonomously judging right from wrong allow her to approach and manage external reality with a gradually declining need for intervention from her parents. When children successfully navigate the developmental tasks of latency, they leave the elementary school years with a sense of confidence in their ability to learn. The grandiosity that, in the preschool years, allowed them to imagine athletic, intellectual, or romantic prowess, is gradually replaced by the capacity to tolerate the frustration that true learning, with all of its failures and false starts, entails. As they actually become more proficient and can manage some of the basic skills such as reading or mathematical calculations that allow them to traffic in the world of adults, they have less need to counteract the humiliation that stems from ignorance and ineptitude with the magical thinking that characterizes early childhood.

The repression of infantile wishes and primitive preoccupations along with identification with parental authority allows, not only for the development of a conscience that both praises and chastises but for meaningful engagement with and manipulation of external reality. The confluence of increased cognitive capacities and emotional maturity facilitates the child's world as it expands to include friends, teachers, and self-reliance as sources of satisfaction. For example, the child who previously had to be escorted to school may now enjoy the companionship of neighborhood children as they all walk to school or safely navigate the route on their bikes.

In order to do the latter, for example, a child must be proficient enough to manage her bicycle reliably without undue attention to the actual physical activity. This, in turn, permits her to attend to the external environment—street signs, traffic, and pedestrians—that may affect her trip to school. Her journey will, doubtless sometimes require her to exercise judgment about issues that concern her safety or pleasure. Perhaps she will discover a short-cut that means going through an isolated area, or maybe other children will suggest an unplanned stop for candy on the way home. Without her actual parents to turn to, she will have to rely on the interaction between her own ego capacities, as she assesses the external realities that affect her physical safety and her conscience, or superego, as she measures the consequences of her actions on her psychological well-being. The interplay of these internal forces will determine her actions. This might result in her deciding that making a stop on the way home would be perfectly safe in addition to a lot of fun. However, knowing that she is to go straight home after school, she may decline the invitation not only because disobedience risks punishment from her parents but out of a recognition that disobedience also risks internally generated anxiety and guilt.

Although latency-age children can indeed rely increasingly on internal agencies to guide their actions, their capacity for judgment is far from infallible. As a newly formed internal agency of authority, the conscience of a young latency child can easily succumb to the voice of external authority. This leaves children, who are competent enough to make their way in the world without always being under the watchful eye of their parents particularly vulnerable to those they view, or who present themselves, as figures to be admired or obeyed. Given this, we shouldn't be surprised that children of this age are often the targets of sexual abuse. It is not simply that they are old enough to have independent, unsupervised contact with scout leaders, teachers, priests or ministers, or other authorities but that they are developmentally susceptible to setting aside their own perceptions or judgments about right and wrong when faced with directives or suggestions from an adult they both admire and fear.

Latency-age children spend much of their time and energy in learning and knowing. Their tenuous but much valued sense of confidence in their own powers of reasoning and judgment can lead to a defensive overconfidence in their knowledge or opinions. This seems to leave children who, like John described below, encounter abuse during latency particularly vulnerable to cognitive confusion in the aftermath of abuse.

John

Over the course of the summer before his 10th birthday, John's parents noticed that their characteristically energetic and outgoing son was unusually somber and moody. During a summer that had included a family vacation and a 2-week stay at overnight camp, John gradually spent more time alone in his room. An extremely bright child who had enjoyed reading and science experiments, John now complained that his books and projects were "boring." John's parents were concerned, but their efforts to talk to John were to no avail. They hoped either that John would "outgrow" whatever was bothering him or that his listlessness would change once he returned to school. However, his fourth-grade teacher found him distractible and a daydreamer who not only didn't complete assignments but couldn't even seem to keep track of what he was supposed to do.

A newsletter from the camp arrived in early fall and caused such anxiety and agitation in John that his parents' bafflement turned to alarm. John's oddly confused and elaborate explanation about why he couldn't return to camp alerted his parents that something must have gone dreadfully wrong there. In response to their gentle but insistent questioning, John eventually revealed that one of his counselors had repeatedly arranged to have John watch while he masturbated to orgasm. During a camping trip John had awakened to find this same counselor in his sleeping bag, with his erect penis pressed against John's buttocks. John lay terrified and confused. Pretending to be asleep, he tried to devise schemes that would prevent a recurrence of his counselor's sexual contacts.

By the time John entered therapy, he had begun, rather successfully, to rewrite his own history to account for the effects of the sexual abuse. He described the dissociative states engendered by his enduring periods of helpless terror as "daydreaming." Unable to tolerate the loss of control that his inability to concentrate engendered, John explained that he was "just kinda lazy." This exceedingly bright child now opined that he had been victimized because he wasn't as smart or as strong as the other kids in his cabin, all of whom he imagined to have prevented the molester's advances.

Having found himself in a very frightening situation that made no sense at all, John did his best to bring his logical powers to the confusion that beset him. The dissociative states that began when John pretended he was "in a tree far, far away," as a means of not attending to his counselor's penis, had a direct effect on John's capacity to concentrate. He felt as if he were in a daydream that he could not escape from. Previously he had known himself as a good student, someone who could learn about and understand the world around him.

When his understanding of himself and his world was pulled out from under him, he reconstructed himself and his world in the context of his developmental concerns. In John's mind, a good student, a smart kid, clearly would not have had this happen to him, so he actually must have been a dumb, weak, lazy kid.

Like many children, John had tried, on his own, to stop the feelings and explain his symptoms away. Though impressive, his efforts were futile precisely because he had tried simply to make the feelings end without really allowing himself to know them and their origins. Obviously, his symptoms stemmed from the molestation, but how exactly did he arrive at those explanations? From what parts of his history and his understanding of the world did he make the particular meanings he did? These are questions that can be answered only with time to listen and reflect. It is true that the process of examining the feelings that he wants so desperately to put aside can cause a child discomfort. Children often try to avoid the pain and disruption of psychotherapy; however, without it, the solutions the child devises on his own are likely to have far more lasting negative consequences.

Latency marks the end of childhood proper, and hence the conclusion of this discussion of development. At the end of the elementary school years children enter preadolescence, marked by the onset of puberty. This serves primarily as a transitory stage, as hormonal changes necessitate concomitant intrapsychic shifts in order to accommodate unfamiliar body sensations and rapid physical growth. That preadolescence is developmentally a kind of limbo is manifested in the ways in which educational systems attempt to manage children in the 12- to 14-year age span. Sometimes sixth-graders are educated in elementary schools, while at other times they are moved into "middle" or "junior high" schools along with seventh- and eighth-graders. In other systems, children remain in elementary schools through the eighth grade, although the older children are designated by privilege and sometimes dress as belonging to the "upper" school. Like the preadolescents themselves, adults often don't know whether to treat these youngsters as children or adolescents. This can leave them particularly vulnerable to sexual predators, who may prey on their childish naiveté while they simultaneously exploit the preadolescent's sexual curiosity.

SUMMARY

I have highlighted some developmental factors that make children particularly vulnerable to abuse at different ages. For example, infants lack the motor skills to move away from an upset parent; their lack of language places great demands on those responsible for understanding and meeting their needs. Toddlers' bids for autonomy, which may express themselves in tantrums or stubbornness, may test the limits of their caregivers' impulse control. The natural sexual interests of pre-schoolers leave them particularly vulnerable to those who would exploit this curiosity for their own needs. The independence accorded children of elementary school may leave them open to abuses of authority by family members, friends, or community figures. This is not to suggest that children are vulnerable to abuse only because of these factors or that theses issues are confined to a single developmental stage. The brief synopsis offered in this chapter is intended as a reminder that we serve our young patients well when we consider the developmental resources, limitations, and concerns they bring to the experience of abuse.

Chapter *Three*

A Template for Developmentally Informed Evaluations

We observe behavior far more easily than we can analyze it. The child's very entrance into our office gives us our first clues about her vision of the world and the concerns she brings to us. When viewed from a developmentally informed perspective, the manner in which a child approaches and uses, or resists and avoids, a new space often provides extremely important information about the child and her attempts to manage both internally generated tasks and externally imposed hardships. Like standardized tests that allow the observer to compare the responses of many children to the same stimuli, the relative constancy of the therapist's playroom or office provides an ideal context for initial observations of a child's relationship to her physical environment and the people in it.

I offer the two following vignettes to demonstrate the richness of information that can be gained when a child's movements, or stillness, in a room are considered in a developmentally informed context. Often, more than words, the child's behavior offers insight into the *child's* perspective on the world. Children's interests in entering into or avoiding psychotherapy often differ from the reasons adults give for bringing them. Sometimes they articulate their views: "I'm not coming here because there's nothing wrong with me," or "I need to talk to someone because I'm too scared to go to camp and my mom says I have to go anyway." At other times, only our careful attention to children's interactions with us, including their use of the environment we provide, tells us what they might want from us or what threats we might pose to their sense of well-being.

In order to illustrate some of the unique perspectives developmental theory can bring to our evaluation of abused children, in the two cases that follow, I have focused particularly on the children's use of the physical space and the way they manage their proximity to their parents. Especially with preverbal (or, as in these two instances, virtually silent) children, careful observations of their physical behavior may reveal complex stories that will not be reflected in spoken language for many weeks or months.

Amy

Three-year-old Amy was brought for evaluation when her parents discovered that she had been fondled by an older neighbor boy who sometimes stayed with Amy for brief periods while her mother ran errands. He had been one of her favorite playmates.

Amy was sitting in her mother's lap when I greeted them in the waiting room. She looked at me suspiciously; with thumb in mouth and blanket in hand she followed me slowly to the office, one step behind and firmly attached to her mother. Upon entering the office she went immediately to the dollhouse, where she played quietly for most of the session. She had positioned herself in close proximity to her mother but across the room from me. By burying her head in the dollhouse, she kept her back planted solidly toward me. From this outpost she gradually engaged her mother in her doll play, handing her dolls to dress and undress. After a bit, as she turned to her mother, she would steal glances over her shoulder in my direction. As the first session drew to a close, she felt brave enough to turn completely around and give me a careful inspection.

Amy began the next session from the same position. However, within a few minutes she moved some of the dolls and furniture out of the house, arranging them so that she faced me as she played. After a few more minutes I commented on how carefully she was looking at me and all of the new things around her. She nodded and extended a doll to me. This move required me to move closer in order to accept her offer. Amy's choreography of this session resulted in her positioning herself between her mother and me. She busied herself with the dolls, moving freely between the two of us.

To begin to understand Amy's behavior in these two sessions, we need to consider the developmental tasks confronting her. Amy was just 3 when she was brought for evaluation. She had only recently started attending a preschool program two mornings a week. By her mother's report, both she and Amy had initially found the separation difficult, but over the last weeks Amy had begun eagerly to anticipate school mornings and her mother to look forward to her free time.

Her mother described Amy as a generally happy child who liked "being the boss" and enjoyed playing with other children. However, Amy's behavior had changed significantly in the few days since the molestation. Since then, Amy had been fearful and fretful, clinging to her mother whenever they left the house. She refused to attend nursery school.

So, in the days prior to her arrival at my office, Amy had dealt with a number of new children and adults at nursery school. She had been molested by a "friend," a child whom she had previously trusted. As a consequence, she had been taken to the sexual abuse clinic where she underwent a physical examination by a pediatrician who, though skilled and sensitive, was unfamiliar to her. Amy was then interviewed by a worker from Child Protective Services before arriving on my doorstep to face yet another stranger!

Naturally, then, Amy initially showed no desire to interact with me. In fact, she made it clear, from her behavior, that she did not want me anywhere near her—either physically or verbally. Even though Amy's mother indicated by both her words and actions that I was someone to be trusted, Amy remained staunch in her suspicions. Her insistence on maintaining close physical proximity to her mother was a definite regression from the pleasure she had enjoyed in going off on her own only a few days earlier.

How do we understand Amy's behavior in a developmental context? First of all, as a preschooler, Amy's newly acquired sense of autonomy and independence had recently been tested by her entry into nursery school. After some initial hesitation, she had demonstrated her capacity successfully to negotiate the nursery-school world of new toys and people without her mother's companionship. Relying on her teachers as substitutes, Amy showed the resiliency necessary for playing and sharing with other children. Her capacity for language and tolerance for delay enabled her to meet the demands of an externally imposed schedule and to move freely from structured to unstructured activities.

Just as she had at the beginning of nursery school, when she came to my office, Amy turned to her mother for comfort in an unfamiliar situation. A securely attached 3-year-old typically uses a parent as a "home base" when confronting new people or places. So Amy's behavior upon entering my office easily falls within developmental norms for a child of her age. However, her staying by her mother's side for an entire 50 minutes alerts us to Amy's anxiety, particularly when we know from her mother that she has previously separated readily to go to nursery school. Now she will not look around a new room even in her mother's presence and with her mother's encouragement.

Although we can form a number of hypotheses about the meaning of Amy's behavior, we must also be cautious about drawing overly broad conclusions from our initial observations. For example, we cannot conclude from Amy's behavior that she lacks curiosity about me, the office, or the toys beyond the dollhouse. Given her recent trauma, she may have restricted her curiosity about the world beyond the safe mother; curiosity can lead to exploration and in some cases, as Amy unfortunately learned, to harm. On the other hand, she may be intensely interested but too frightened to allow herself to explore.

Happily these initial observations indicate that, at least in this context, Amy's regression has not been severe. She does not crawl into her mother's lap or bury her face in her mother's clothing. She does not cry, and her demeanor does not suggest severe fright. Although Amy shows no interest in talking with me, she does not interrupt when her mother and I talk; that is, she asks for her mother's attention in appropriate ways. She engages her in doll play and tolerates sharing her attention, at least for short periods. Note also the behavioral shifts from the first to the second session. Amy remembers me and the office; by behaving in a less cautious manner, she demonstrates her ability to act on her assessment that she is not in imminent danger.

Amy's staying in close proximity to her mother serves as quite an adaptive response to the recent events in her life. She returns to the safety and security her mother's presence offers. This dependence on a reliable other suggests that Amy is conscious of her anxiety. Turning to the familiarity of a loving parent in a new situation is certainly preferable to her relying on defensive strategies that attempt to mask, rather than express, her feelings. For example, if Amy had adopted a pseudomature stance or counterphobically approached this strange situation and unfamiliar person with unwarranted friendliness, we might wonder if she was at all aware of her anxiety or whether this behavior was successfully keeping her intense feelings out of conscious awareness.

About 1 year later, when moving to a new school, Amy again began to cling to her mother and to express numerous fears. Her mother had expected some regression but not the intensity of anxiety that Amy seemed to be feeling. This time when Amy, now 4 years old, arrived for a visit, she greeted me warmly in the waiting room and proudly announced that she remembered the way to my office. She asked about the dollhouse as we walked down the hall together, ahead of her mother. Once in the office, she quickly went to the dollhouse but after a few minutes began to explore other toys, noting what she remembered and what seemed unfamiliar.

Again, focusing on Amy's relationship to her physical environment, we see that her development has continued nicely over the intervening year. She is now open and expansive; she remembers a friendly environment and responds accordingly. Although her behavior may be regressed in the unfamiliarity of the new school situation, the symptom has not generalized. Had Amy behaved this way on our first meeting, we would have wondered about her lack of caution. One year later, her free and relaxed relationship to the physical space is reassuring. She "feels at home."

Jim

Jim's father initiated the evaluation of his 10-year-old son because of his concern that Jim seemed completely unable to separate from his mother. He felt that Jim was too dependent on his mother, whom he described as "babying" her only son.

Jim's parents were divorced; his father's weekend visits had gradually diminished over the previous months as Jim expressed increasing anxiety about being away from his mother. In the 2 weeks prior to the father's contacting me, Jim had refused to leave the house, although he seemed content to see his father as long as his mother was nearby.

The mother corroborated the father's report of Jim's behavior. However, her explanations differed from the father's. She thought Jim was afraid to be alone with his father, whom she described as having a wicked temper. Though Jim had not complained of being hit, she wondered if that might have happened. She felt quite certain that the father had yelled at Jim, since he "screams at everyone else." She said she encouraged Jim to go with his father, but he simply refused to leave the house.

When I greeted Jim and his mother in the waiting room, I noticed that a table that normally sat between two chairs had been moved from its usual place so that the chairs could be placed side by side. Jim and his mother occupied those seats. Jim looked panicked at my entrance to the room and grabbed his mother's arm. I invited them to the office; Jim waited for his mother to move, then, clinging to her hand, walked so closely behind her that she nearly tripped over his feet. In the office, he sat in a chair with her, even though it was a warm day and they were too large for both to fit comfortably into this space. The physical discomfort this caused both of them was obvious.

After about 15 minutes, during which time Jim had not spoken a word, his mother reminded him that she was planning to return to the waiting room, where she would remain until the end of the session. Jim vigorously shook his head "no" and tightened his grip on her arm. The mother tried, initially gently and in a reassuring tone, to move away. When this was clearly impossible, she suggested with some irritation that since she was quite warm and cramped sharing a chair with him, she would, at least, move to another chair. Jim tightened his grip with a defiant look in my direction. I commented that his concern about allowing any distance at all between himself and his mother was very clear.

Jim's mother complained about this behavior, noting that she couldn't go out with friends or even to the grocery store without Jim putting up a fuss. She was getting tired of having to walk him to school. Angrily she announced that it had to stop. She simply would not stand for being controlled by a 10-year-old, especially since she had recently met a man at work who liked to go out dancing, an activity that she had sorely missed since her divorce. Jim continued his angry stare in my direction. His mother sighed and settled into the chair; she chatted about her work and told me a bit about Jim's new school. His mother worried that Jim's grades were slipping because of frequent absences. At his old school, they hadn't really paid too much attention to lateness or absences. She wondered if Jim didn't like the new school because it was too strict. Jim said nothing.

At the time of the second scheduled session, I opened my office door to find Jim and his mother standing at the top of the stairs, both panting and sweating profusely. Jim was silently and angrily yanking on his mother's arm as she desperately clung to the railing to avoid being dragged down the stairs. She explained, as best she could under the circumstances, that Jim had not wanted to come to the session and that she had quite literally dragged him up the stairs to the office. Since Jim was a rather large 10-year-old and the stairway was quite tall, this would have been quite a feat.

However, when Jim gave a final tug, his mother sighed and with an air of resignation said that it just didn't seem that an evaluation would do much good right now. They walked down the stairs, hand in hand. Jim complained that he was hot and sweaty. His mother eventually agreed that they could go somewhere for a soda before heading home.

Jim's behavior is obviously very troubling. Like the baby who feels comfortable exploring the world only from the safety of the mother's arms, Jim insists that his mother stay within his reach—in fact, he was unwilling to venture farther than arm's length in the two episodes just described. Although it can be difficult to look beyond the controlling aspects of Jim's clinging, this child is paying a very high price to stay so close to his mother. He is not quite literally sitting in his mother's lap in the waiting room, but Jim's proximity to her and his demeanor both indicate that he feels unable to bear any physical or psychological distance between them. Jim demonstrates absolutely no interest in the environment beyond his mother, except as a potential threat to his hold on her. His panic when I entered the waiting room suggests a child terrified of any separation.

A developmental consideration of these brief observations makes abundantly clear why, intuitively, we should be gravely concerned about Jim's initial responses to a new environment, including the therapist. The developmental tasks confronting Jim require, in large measure, the capacity to turn his attention to the world beyond his immediate family.

We must wonder about the causes of Jim's unwillingness to separate from his mother. He has just began attending a new school, which might cause some anxiety, perhaps a lot, but not enough to account for the dramatic behavior in my office or that described by his parents. Even though he may be unaccustomed to his new school,

Jim is 10 years old and by now has had 4 or 5 years of practice in adapting to new teachers, students, and, presumably, increasing demands for independent work. If all is going reasonably well developmentally, we would expect Jim to look to teachers and friends for gratification and praise rather than to retreat into a seemingly unbreakable bond with his mother.

In general, 10-year-olds do not want to spend all of their time with their mothers. In fact, they tend to complain when they feel their time with friends or for activities they consider fun or important are impinged upon by parents' demands on their time and attention. From this vantage, point it is clear that Jim's inability to separate from his mother would severely interfere with his mastery of developmental tasks. It's very hard to play ball with your friends while holding on to your mother's hand!

Again, we must be cautious about drawing overly broad conclusions about the motivations for and meanings of Jim's behavior. We don't know whether his lack of curiosity about me and the office is apparent or actual. He may inhibit his curiosity out of a fear that if he diverts his attention from his mother she may likewise direct her attention away from him and toward her new boyfriend. Alternatively, he may be so intensely preoccupied with his mother that he actually takes little notice of the world beyond her. Regardless of the reasons for Jim's restricted relationship to his physical environment, his behavior is a matter for concern because of the severity of the inhibitory regression.

It would worry us less if, for example, Jim could engage his mother in any kind of play, whether a game or playful verbal interchange. If, when she mentions her boyfriend, he were critical of him or verbally demonstrated some competitiveness with this intruder, we would find reassurance in Jim's capacity to use language to formulate and express his feelings. Because he doesn't speak, we can only wonder whether Jim consciously articulates his reasons for demanding such physical closeness to his mother or, instead, only feels intense, inexplicable anxiety when out of her presence.

By the second session, Jim has intensified his efforts to remain close to his mother, this time successfully prohibiting either of them from having contact with the therapist. This suggests that Jim does not feel a sense of safety in my office or with me. Indeed it poses such danger that he cannot even bear to enter.

We learn nothing about the suggestion that Jim's behavior is motivated by a fear of his father. Jim has not complained to his mother about being hit; his mother speculates that her ex-husband may yell at his son. Jim may indeed be afraid of his father, or his mother may be projecting her feelings onto Jim. Jim's insistence on seeing his father only in his mother's company seems to coincide with his mother's developing a new relationship. We might wonder if a wish to reunite his parents motivates Jim's behavior.

From such limited data, we can only speculate about the complex conscious and unconscious interactions between Jim and his parents that have resulted in this child's almost being imprisoned by his need to remain near his mother. For the mother's part, although she complains, she acquiesces to his every demand. The mother's comment that an evaluation "might not do any good right now" overtly conveys her opinion that the therapist is as powerless as she in the face of Jim's demands. She may also covertly be sending the more powerful message that she, herself, is so terrified of separation that she is willing to allow her son to become emotionally impaired rather than confront whatever anxieties their mutual dependence masks.

As this clinical material illustrates, sometimes the child's most salient communication comes in his silence, his unwillingness to reveal himself in either words or action. The child's unrehearsed interactions with us, whether conscious or unconscious, will ultimately prove most useful in our therapeutic work. If we set the agenda or ply him with our questions or those suggested by others we lose the opportunity to discover what he finds important. Although data about the child's background can often inform us about the issues that bring the child to us for help, data can obscure as well as inform.

When we feel pressured to query the child about the external details of his life, we suggest that such matters are privileged over his feelings, fantasies, and the material he generates from within himself, rather than in response to an externally generated agenda. Particularly in our treatment of abused children, the temptation to focus on the abusive history can be very great. Parents, teachers, attorneys, and investigators may all have a stake in our discovering the details of an abusive past. Or they may urge us to raise the issue with the child so that we might see and evaluate his reaction. This ultimately may be a crucial activity (see Chapters 5 and 10), but undue focus on the issues that adults find important will interfere with our quiet attention to and acceptance of the concerns the child brings to us.

An evaluation must begin with the gathering of information. In my experience, the longer we can listen patiently, directing our comments and questions specifically to the child's words and actions, the more we will learn about the child and the part(s) we may be asked to play in the psychological drama she brings to our office.

If, for example, rather than asking a child how she does in school, we attend to the mixture of complexity and concreteness in her language, the form and content of her expression or inhibition of curiosity, her attitudes toward winning and losing, the skills she brings and the difficulty of the games or activities she suggests, her capacity to move between fantasy and reality, and the affective world she introduces into the therapeutic relationship, we will likely have a great deal of insight into the child's academic performance, as well as her relationships with teachers and peers. Furthermore, such information requires no corroboration; it is equally available to both therapist and child.

This is not to discount the very real value of the perspectives that parents, teachers, counselors, or others can and do offer child therapists; we would be foolish and inefficient to undertake our work without making use of these resources or to remain ignorant of the child's medical history, school performance, or family constellation. However, this information, like that the child gives in response to our questions, is of a different order and serves a different purpose than does the material she spontaneously produces. The former provide the background for the therapeutic work; the latter make it come alive.

Perhaps particularly in work with abused children, there is a sensed mandate, both internally and externally generated, for the therapist to "cure," to apply a poultice that will once-and-for-all extract the child's pain from her being and her future—to assert our expertise over the demons that torment her. When we fall victim to this very seductive temptation, we risk trying to demonstrate the efficacy of our learning at the expense of tolerating our ignorance. There is a delicate and probably impossible balance to be maintained between holding to a theory that will prevent both therapist and patient from drowning in the morass of chaos and uncertainty that surrounds child abuse on the one hand and, on the other hand, setting aside our theories in order to sink into the affective chasm that characterizes abuse. Approaching our work in the spirit of reflection and humility may allow us to maintain a sense of integrity as we struggle against the limits of our knowledge in our work with abused children.

Chapter Four

Neurobiology and Psychology: The Formation and Meaning of Symptoms

Any discussion of clinical work with children who have withstood the pain, terror, and confusion of sexual or physical abuse demonstrates clearly that these are not easy children to treat. Indeed, their symptoms often make it difficult for others just to be with them for a short time. Bobby screams and hits at the slightest provocation. Rosa flirts with her male counselors and seductively rubs against them. A pleasant conversation with Ellen suddenly erupts into a vicious verbal assault when her therapist misunderstands something she has said. José stiffens with terror at any sudden noise. Suzy tells her attorney that her father touched her with his penis; a week later she says she *did not* say that and accuses the attorney of being a liar. Jack seems preoccupied; when his teacher asks him to repeat an instruction, he can't remember what she just said.

Extended, thoughtful exploration of the symptoms displayed by each of these children will undoubtedly reveal powerful and important unconscious meanings and motivations. The meanings will be determined largely by the individual child's constitutional factors, developmental history, and prior and current relationships. However, symptomatic behavior also has profoundly important neurological underpinnings;

some symptom clusters, such as disregulation of affect, behavioral disorganization, or extreme difficulties in interpersonal relationships, do repeatedly occur in our observations of abused children. This suggests that the similarities among these children may arise from abuse-inflicted neurological deviations, while the differences arise from the uniqueness of personal history.

To be most effective in understanding or treating a child who has been abused, we must consider this complex interplay of psychological and physiological forces. If we attend only to the impact on the brain or only the effects on the mind, we will falsify the inevitable interconnectedness of the two and diminish our appreciation of the child's experience (Grigsby & Schneiders, 1991; Green, 1995; Dubowitz, Black, Harrington, & Verschoore, 1993). We take for granted that a blow to a child's head may inflict temporary or permanent damage to the brain and that a rape may cause lasting vaginal or rectal scarring. However, when examining the effects of trauma from the perspectives of neurobiology, endocrinology, and psychophysiology, we see the research repeatedly and convincingly demonstrates that the child's brain itself need not be directly assaulted nor the child's genitals permanently scarred for serious damage to occur (Brown, 1991; George, 1996; Krystal, 1978, 1991; Lawrence, Cozolino, & Foy, 1995; Schaaf & McCanne, 1994; Toth & Cicchetti, 1996).

At the same time, aggressive and sexual assaults affect not only children's brains but their minds. Psychological changes make it difficult for them to trust, love, learn, or remember. When a child can't learn, he may think that there is something wrong with his brain, that he is stupid. If he has been abused, there may indeed be something wrong with his brain, leaving him not only feeling stupid, but possibly behaving stupidly, as well. When a child has been sexually assaulted, particularly if assaulted by someone she trusted, she may feel that it was *her* sexuality that provoked this contact. Indeed, if her consequent behavior becomes more sexualized, she may well find herself increasingly the object of sexual attention. She may then erroneously take this attention as confirmation of her belief that she was responsible for the initial seduction.

At times of dramatic developmental changes—adolescence, pregnancy, or menopause, for example—we easily link the psychological with the physiological. It would be not only foolish but demeaning to consider an adolescent's rapidly fluctuating mood swings without taking into account the enormous hormonal changes that characterize this period of life. It would be equally foolhardy to ignore the profoundly conflicting emotional needs of the adolescent who is neither child nor adult and who simultaneously wishes and tries to be both.

Although psychodynamic clinicians are disposed toward seeing irrational or perplexing behavior as arising from physiological processes at times of significant developmental crises, we have not always given equal attention to the physiological crises emanating from abusive experiences during childhood. This is curious because we clearly acknowledge the extraordinary emotional impact these assaults can have on a child. This inconsistency may derive from our inclination to privilege interventions that we do understand over those that we do not; like the surgeon who does not immediately consider acupuncture as a viable treatment or the osteopath who does not look to synthetic drugs for cure, we are bound by our education and training.

Our wish to deny the impact of abuse on physiological processes may also emerge out of a fear of seeing the child as permanently or irreparably damaged. Despite what we know, we may harbor a wish to relegate the effects of abuse solely to the world of individually created meaning, that is, to view the child's symptoms as arising only from unconscious conflict or interpersonal strife. If we fail to appreciate that these symptoms represent a lack or a disruption of reliable neural pathways, we may tend toward a potentially dangerous impatience with the pervasive and lasting quality of the child's symptomatic behavior. Along with his caregivers and teachers, we may overestimate the child's capacity for independent decision or action, falsely assuming that insight or understanding will offer the child sufficient tools for changing her behavior and affective responses. Even elementary knowledge about the neurological underpinnings of symptoms such as distractibility, hyper- or hyposensitivities, agitation, aggression, or memory lapses that commonly arise from physical and sexual abuse deepens our understanding of the work required of a child struggling to recover from their traumatic effects. Such knowledge also increases our effectiveness as consultants when we are called upon to assist teachers and caregivers in helping these most troubled and difficult children.

Our understandings of the effects of child abuse influence aspects of our therapeutic work from the macrosphere of consultation with teachers, tutors, or school counselors to the microsphere of our direct comments within the therapeutic relationship. Consider, for example, the theoretical underpinnings and the meanings of different comments to a child about the motivation for his inappropriately aggressive behavior.

> "Sometimes you get scared of the kids on the playground because you're afraid they're going to beat you up, just like your father did."

> "Sometimes you get so scared that you can't think, and the whole world seems like a dangerous place."

> "When you feel scared, your brain runs so fast that you can't think about whether you're really in danger or not."

All of these statements speak to the child's underlying fear, but they offer different admixtures of psychological and physiological explanations to the child.

Even a basic grasp of the neurophysiological effects of abuse expands the resources we bring to psychotherapy. Below I have sketched a very rudimentary framework for understanding neurobiological responses to trauma. I offer this outline as an introduction to considerations of both the impact of abuse and the effects of psychotherapy on the structures underlying behavior. An understanding of the complex functions of the brain must begin with a grasp of the structure and mechanisms of the brain. Therefore, I first highlight some pertinent aspects of normative neuroanatomy, the function of neurotransmitters, brain development, and the interrelated structural aspects of memory and affect regulation. I then turn to aspects of memory, affect, and attachment that are so vital to healthy development and so frequently disrupted when children suffer sexual or physical abuse.

The nervous system, with the brain at its center, is uniquely designed to gather, assess, store information and initiate the action that maintains and preserves the human organism (Coen, 1985; Nolte, 1989; Rakic, 1991). Whether sensing changes in temperature and responding by altering the body's metabolic rate, alerting the body to cross the street to avoid a potentially dangerous situation, or conveying love and affection to another through language and action, the nervous system is an exquisitely designed communication system. Communication within the nervous system depends on both electrical and chemical processes. Electrical impulses move information within cells, while neurochemicals are responsible for conveying information from one cell to another.

CELLS OF THE NERVOUS SYSTEM

This elaborate communication network depends on *neurons*, the irregularly shaped nerve cells that comprise about 10% of the billions of cells in the human nervous system. *Sensory neurons* collect information from the body's internal and external environment, *interneurons* transmit information, and *motor neurons* activate the muscles of the body. In general, each neuron consists of a *cell body*, an *axon* protruding from one point, and masses of *dendrites* extending from the other points of the cell body. The dendrites receive information, which then, via electrical conduction, passes through the cell body into the axon, the point at which information is transmitted from that cell to others.

Glial cells, which enhance and protect the neurons, account for the other 90% of cells in the nervous system. These cells are of particular importance during certain *critical periods* of neural development. During these "preset" times of rapid growth, different neural pathways become highly *myelinated*, that is, the individual axons in a particular cluster become coated with myelin, a fatty substance contained in some glial cells. This sheath, laid down in a spiral pattern, speeds the conduction of electrical impulses through the axon, thus enhancing the efficiency of the individual neuron and developing the pathway in which it participates. For example, neurons in the visual cortex undergo a period of increased myelination 2 to 3 months postnatally (Schore, 1997), while language tracts become highly developed between 2 and 3 years postnatally, or during the period when children typically enjoy the most rapid acquisition of language.

BRAIN ANATOMY

The example of the human brain that we most frequently see depicted in drawings or models usually represents the adult brain. A familiar illustration of the brain may include labels of different areas of the cortex according to specialization, for example showing Broca's area, which controls expressive language and Wernicke's area, the center of language comprehension. This many inadvertently lead us to imagine the brain as made up of fixed structures. Especially when considering the infant brain, which is not well differentiated, it is more accurate to think of the brain as composed of anatomical potentials, shaped by experience. Indeed neurological development involves the process of increasing specialization of neural tracts and cortical centers. While abuse has the potential for complex effects on multiple, interrelated aspects of brain centers and functions (including language comprehension and expression), the anatomical outline below intends to highlight the parts of the brain most crucial to attachment, memory, and affect regulation, that is, those areas apparently most vulnerable to neurological disruption in the wake of abuse.

The anatomy of the human brain reflects the way it has grown and changed over millions of years, not in an organized process, but through evolutionary pathways that sometimes added new structures and sometimes put old elements to new uses. The oldest and most primitive part of the brain is the *brain stem*, sometimes referred to as the "reptilian brain" because of its similarity to the entire brain of reptiles. The brainstem controls the vital functions necessary for survival. From this area arise regulation of respiration and heart rate. For the purposes of this discussion, it is important to note the role of the brainstem in receiving information about impending dangers and controlling various states of arousal. The states of hyperarousal related to "fight or flight" patterns originate in the brainstem.

At the rear of the brainstem lies the *cerebellum*. This is the center of control over posture, balance, and coordination of the habitual muscular movements involved in activities such as walking, sitting, smiling, or grimacing. The cerebellum has a "motoric memory," which allows us to repeat learned movements without conscious thought. We do not think about how to smile, or sit, or stand. The cerebellum pilots our movements as we approach a bicycle, straddle it, and pedal off, even if we have not ridden a bike for months or years.

Of great importance to our discussion is the *limbic system*, sometimes referred to as the "mammalian brain" because it is highly developed in mammals. It consists of a ring of tissue that sits between the brainstem and the cortex. As its name suggests, the limbic system is not a single structure but an array of related structures including the hippocampus, the amygdala, the pituitary gland, thalamus, and hypothalamus.

The *hypothalamus* is perhaps the most crucial part of the limbic system; it regulates heart rate, hunger, thirst, sleep, waking, blood

pressure, and sexual drives. It also controls the endocrine, or hormonal, system through communication with the *pituitary gland*, the body's
master gland. Emotional expression also originates in the hypothalamus.

The *amygdala* plays an important role in the subjective experience
of feeling states, particularly fear and aggression. The *thalamus* has a
crucial role in our capacity to make not only cognitively determined
but affectively based discriminations. Even if we could absorb all of
the information that besets us from moment to moment, we have no
need of every sensation or perception that impinges on our nervous
system. The thalamus functions as a control center for sorting the
millions of discrete pieces of internal and external data continually
bombarding us; some pieces of information are transmitted to other
parts of the brain for processing or storage, while others are inhibited
in their journey. The *hippocampus* is crucial in both short- and long-
term memory. With its multitudes of neuronal connections to both
lower brain structures and the neocortex, the hippocampus appears to
process stimuli and deliver those percepts destined for storage in
long-term memory to appropriate areas of the frontal cortex.

The extent of the influence of trauma on the limbic system should
be evident when we consider the functions of this area of the brain in
relationship to symptoms, such as hyperarousal, unmodulated affective
responses, flashbacks, and disruption of attention, associated with
trauma. However, emotional responsiveness, like most neural activity,
is not confined to a single area of the brain. The limbic system is
intimately connected with cortical centers, particularly with the *orbital
frontal cortex*, which is "uniquely involved in social and emotional
behaviors and in the homeostatic regulation of body and motivational
states" (Schore, 1997).

In the familiar illustrations or models mentioned above, the
cerebral cortex, with its array of convolutions and fissures resulting from
its being repeatedly folded in upon itself, is evident because it is the
uppermost and outermost aspect of the brain. The cortex covers the
largest part of the brain—the *cerebrum*, divided laterally into two
hemispheres that are connected by the *corpus callosum*, the largest
pathway of nerve fibers in the brain. In general, the *right hemisphere*
controls the left side of the body and the *left hemisphere* controls the
right side. However, the hemispheres are not mirror images of each
other. Each hemisphere contains areas of specialization not found in
the other. In the adult brain, the multitude of pathways contained in

the corpus callosum allows for different aspects of information to be spread through and retrieved from various areas of the cerebral cortex. Thus, a single experience will both activate and be "acted upon" by many cortical centers while simultaneously inhibiting the actions of other pathways. Because of functional specialization, both hemispheres participate in complex processes as symbolic thought, language, and art. Indeed, the interplay of the varying functions of the two hemispheres enlivens and enriches these uniquely human activities.

The cerebral cortex or "gray matter," the most highly evolved portion of the brain, gets its characteristic color from the cell bodies and dendrites of the billions of neurons originating in it. When we consider that the dendrites are the parts of nerve cells designed to receive data, the importance of the cortex in processing and synthesizing internally and externally generated stimuli becomes clear. In addition to being divided into two hemispheres, the cerebral cortex is characterized by four functional, interconnected lobes. The *occipital lobe*, or visual cortex, lies at the rear and base of the two hemispheres. The auditory cortex is part of the *temporal lobe*, situated near each temple. In addition to hearing, the temporal lobes are also associated with perception and memory. The *parietal lobes*, located between the occipital and frontal lobes, are associated with language and the ability to maintain orientation to time and space. The *frontal lobes*, found just behind the forehead, are the largest of the four cortical lobes and are intimately connected with the limbic system. The frontal lobe functions as a control center for the brain. Planning, judgment, decision making, personality, and the regulation of psychological and biological states emanate from the frontal lobe. Current research increasingly points to the importance of the orbital frontal lobe as crucial in determining and regulating the emotional and social aspects of behavior (Schore, 1994).

NEUROTRANSMITTERS

Neurological processes, the sending and receiving of information and the development and maintenance of pathways for conveying information, depend on the chemical conduction of signals from one neuron to another. Neurotransmitters emanate from the axon of one neuron and cross a synapse, or gap, to the receptor cells on the dendrites of other neurons. The message is then relayed, via the same process, to still other neurons until it reaches its final destination. Millions of neurons are involved in the processing of even a single, discrete piece of information, which means that any bit of information may be conveyed to many parts of the nervous system for processing or storage. Although a neuronal transmission might terminate at cells quite distant from the brain, resulting in the activation or inhibition of motor activity or glandular secretion, the vast majority of neuronal transmissions terminate in other neurons (Solomon, 1985).

When a neurotransmitter is released into a synaptic cleft, the space between the axon of one neuron and the dendrites of another, it must lock onto a receptor site specifically designed to accept it before it can affect the receiving neuron. Just as a lock is designed to accept only keys of a particular shape, receptor sites will accept only particular neurotransmitters. However, unlike a house with a single lock on a single door, neurons are like houses with multitudes of doors—opening some will excite the activities within the house, while opening others will calm the activity. Whether a neuron is activated/excited or inhibited/calmed depends on which "doors" are unlocked by given neurotransmitters. The activation or inhibition of a neuronal pathway may depend on the unlocking of a certain, critical number of doors—even though some receptor sites are filled, that number may be insufficient to affect the pathway. In other cases, there may be an oversupply of a given neurotransmitter; perhaps too many doors or houses are unlocked, and the entire "neighborhood" becomes either overly excited or cannot be roused.

The primary neurotransmitters pertinent to our discussion are serotonin and the catacholamines, dopamine and norepinephrine. These play critical roles in the expression and regulation of mood, learning, memory, and stress response. Dopamine and norepinephrine are important mood regulators; lowered levels are associated with depression. Serotonin plays a critical role in the maintenance of mood and induction of sleep; lowered levels of serotonin have been associated with mood disorders and schizophrenia. The availability of different neurotransmitters is not static but varies in response to changes in factors such as diet, sleep/wake patterns, exercise, internal and external stimulation, and interpersonal relationships.

The crucial role of these neurochemicals in normal brain development and function, as well as symptomatic response to and recovery from trauma, cannot be overlooked. Indeed, the vast majority of psychotropic medications developed to treat mental illness—that is, to regulate mood and its attendant behavior—derive their effect by artificially enhancing or limiting the synaptic availability of these neurotransmitters. In general, psychotropic medications affect the brain in one of three ways.

- Some medications are synthetic copies of the body's own neurotransmitters that are accepted by the receptor sites of the target cells. They can either enhance the action of the neurotransmitter, by increasing the available pool of messengers or block its action by acting merely as "placeholders" that fill the receptor site but lack the chemical properties to affect the cell.
- Other medications affect the chemical processes that either synthesize or destroy the neurotransmitters—thereby either increasing or decreasing their availability as messengers.
- A third type of medications affect the brain's "recycling" of neurotransmitters. When neurotransmitters are released into the synaptic cleft, those that do not bind to a receptor site are reabsorbed by the axons that discharged them. Those that are reabsorbed are temporarily inactivated. If a medication "blocks the reuptake" of a neurotransmitter, it makes more of that chemical messenger available. For example, depression has been correlated with a decrease in serotonin levels. Therefore, medications that block the reuptake of serotonin, that is, make more serotonin available in the synaptic clefts, can help to alleviate depression.

BRAIN DEVELOPMENT

Anatomically, the human brain contains the phylogenetically and genetically determined scaffolding for the reception, processing, and storage of information from the environment. Although the full complement of nerve cells is present at birth, massive cerebral development and growth take place postnatally, particularly during the first 2 years of life. The form of this growth will depend, not only on the genetic make-up of the individual but on the particular environment in which the baby lives and grows. Neither the child's brain nor her environment is static; each exerts reciprocal influences on the other. Therefore, even if we could know precisely the unique genetic predispositions contained in any infant's mind, because neurological development and experience are intimately connected, it is no more possible to know precisely the microstructures that will be built on the inborn scaffolding than it is to predict the events in any child's future.

The importance of this concept simply cannot be overstated—a child's brain is in a state of constant flux, continually altering and adapting to its internal and external environment. This must be taken into account in any developmental assessment of the impact of trauma; the brain (and mind) of a child who has enjoyed an optimal environment prior to a single abusive incident will be quite different from that of a child who has suffered early deprivation or who lives in a state of chronic emotional, physical, or sexual abuse. Just as we would expect an otherwise healthy child to recover from a flu more easily than a child whose immune system is already compromised in some important ways, common sense tells us that some children will recover from the effects of abuse more readily and completely than others. Thus we must assess not only the impact of the trauma on current neurobiological development, but we must consider the neurological substrate laid down in earlier developmental periods.

At the infant's birth, most of his cerebral nerve cells have relatively few dendritic spines, the neurons' finger-like receptors. Thus, neurologically, the young infant is ill equipped to absorb the massive amounts of internal and external stimuli bombarding his immature system. At predetermined times, or critical periods, different nerve tracts, groups of neurons and projections clustered according to function, undergo massive proliferation of dendrites. Both individually and as working groups, they become increasingly receptive to particular kinds of information. During these critical periods, the myelination of axons also promotes neurological growth. As described above, when wrapped in the fatty sheath of myelin provided by glial cells, axons become more efficient conductors of information, thus increasing the potential for the release of neurotransmitters to the proliferating dendrites.

This postnatal neurological development creates and enhances the neural pathways necessary for the transmission of information to specific processing and storage sites. For example, the corpus collosum, which, in the adult, distributes information within the right and left hemispheres of the cortex, is very rudimentary in the infant. This means that incoming information impinges more-or-less equally on both hemispheres because the specific distribution pathways have not been established. Neurological channels are built through use—particularly during critical developmental periods. Paths that are well used will become larger and more stable, while those that get little use or stimulation may lie dormant or disappear. Imagine a large grassy area between a school and a housing development; the children traverse this area along different routes until some pathways become wider and more well defined than others. Because these pathways are easier to travel, they are used more frequently than smaller, less efficient trails, which, gradually, overgrown with grass, are difficult to find. This is similar to the growth of neural pathways. Initially there is an overabundance of dendrites, making numerous pathways available for the transmission of information. Those pathways that receive more stimulation become increasingly efficient, while others are gradually obscured or eliminated.

Thus, we can appreciate the importance of the environment in influencing brain development. Visual stimulation excites and strengthens the visual cortex, just as sounds enhance the development of auditory pathways. Given the human infant's utter helplessness, it should not surprise us that at birth the baby's neurological apparatus is uniquely suited for developing and sustaining the attachments necessary for survival. For example, the newborn's greatest visual acuity sits at approximately 12 inches, or the distance between the nursing infant and her mother's face. Likewise, the young infant's auditory pathways are more responsive to midrange tones, the part of the spectrum into which the human voice falls.

Babies whose caregivers meet their needs for visual, auditory, and tactile stimulation will have a very different experience than those babies who are overstimulated or whose needs are neglected. As the children mature physically, they will make different demands for attention and require different kinds of interaction from those who care for them. All of these experiences will contribute to the unique nature of each individual's neurological development. However, children do not come into the world equally well-endowed. Infants who are neurologically impaired do not process information as easily as neurologically intact infants. Premature infants, babies born drug-addicted, children hampered by illness, birth defects, or genetic conditions are often difficult for caregivers to raise. They may not establish predictable patterns easily, may be difficult to soothe or discipline, or relatively unresponsive to their environment. All of these factors can make the establishment of a positive attachment between children and their caregivers more difficult, thus leaving them more vulnerable to abuse.

From this framework we can turn our attention to three intimately interrelated processes: attachment, affect regulation, and memory. All are essential and can be profoundly affected by physical, sexual, or emotional abuse. It should not be surprising that these are interdependent neurological processes; an environment that facilitates one, benefits all. Traumatic experiences likewise have profound neurological effects, not only on each discreet system, but on the ways they affect each other. Although I have separated them below for the purpose of discussion, in the reality of human lives, both the creation and retrieval of memory are inseparable from our relationships with others and the emotions stirred by those relationships and the events we share. Below I briefly highlight some of the salient aspects of attachment, affect regulation, and memory and consider ways in which physical or sexual abuse may affect each of these critical processes.

DEVELOPMENT AND DISRUPTION
OF ATTACHMENT

Though the neonatal brain is a rather rudimentary organ, as we have seen from the above discussion, it is uniquely primed to sustain and enhance the life of the organism. At birth, survival depends on the brain's capacity to regulate the body's vital functions such as breathing, heart rate, and temperature. However, the continuing life of the human infant also absolutely depends on interaction with the environment (Young, 1985; Noshpitz & King, 1991). She can do nothing for herself and must rely on the mother, or her substitute, for care. Neurologically, the infant is organized, not only to receive the ministrations of her caregivers, but to promote their interest in her. Infant–parent attachment thereby is a reciprocal process, to which both baby and caregiver contribute, though not in equal measure.

While the full-term infant will instinctively root and suck when placed at the breast, someone must either anticipate his hunger or respond appropriately to his cries of distress. Because of the immaturity of the organism, particular to human infants, it is impossible for a baby to seek and find his parent in times of hunger or distress. He must signal his needs vocally and maintain contact through visual engagement. When the "environment," usually the mother, responds to the baby's hungry cry with food, the baby gradually learns that he can deliberately vocalize his needs. Concomitantly, the mother learns to differentiate among her baby's various cries of distress and to minister to the infant accordingly. On one level, this ever-more complex feedback loop of signal-and-response seems so simple and straightforward that it hardly bears mentioning. However, as clinicians interested in the psychology or psychopathology involved in the success or failure of this intricate process, we rarely stop to consider the underlying neurobiological changes that determine the observable behavioral changes in *both* infant and mother.

Because the infant has more to learn and less to draw on, her neurological development in response to interactions will be greater. As axons, dendrites, and the synaptic connections, which allow for the encoding of her experiences, are laid down, the beginning of memory is created. Gradually, the infant has a reservoir of experience arising out of her interaction with the environment. The orbitofrontal cortex, with its multiplicity of connections to lower brain structures as well as other cortical centers, is central to the reciprocal interactions between infant and caregiver that give rise to attachment (Schore, 1994). The attachment-processing connections that are established in infancy significantly influence the behavioral repertoire and affective tone the adult will bring to parenthood and the patterns of attachment she will establish with her own children (Gazzaniga & LeDoux, 1978; Amini et al., 1996; Schore, 1994).

In the wake of trauma, children often exist in a state of hyperarousal, both because of neurophysiological changes and because of a consciously felt need to be alert to potential dangers in the external world. It is not difficult to see how psychological and physiological factors become mutually reinforcing. In a state of hyperarousal, the child is more likely both to notice and to be alarmed by potential threats to her physical safety. A raised voice could be painfully distressing as could an unexpected touch from a teacher or counselor. Because the voice was frightening or the touch uninvited, the child comes to see the people who wish to help her as threatening and providing further evidence that the world truly is a dangerous place, in which one cannot easily rest or feel reassured. The perceived need for hypervigilance is integrated into a feedback loop in which the physiological demands for a state of hyperarousal are increased, thereby making the child more vulnerable to external stimuli. Concomitantly, unless they are attentive to their responses, the adults committed to helping the child may take her responses as a personal rejection. If they withdraw, they diminish her chances for forming new relationships with people on whom she might rely for soothing and comfort. Paradoxically, the more bereft and despairing the child becomes, the more difficult it may be for her to accept the help offered and for those available to offer the help she needs.

Those who work with children who have been abused know the tension that can arise if a child routinely hears the slightest rise in our tone of voice as intimidation, or responds to a casual movement (Person & Klar, 1994) as a physical threat. We may understandably withdraw or become overly cautious in words and actions, both to protect ourselves and the child. In this way, the abused child's inability to regulate affect can perpetuate patterns of abusive attachment.

When a child's early attachments are indiscriminate—that is, he has simply been unable to form a primary attachment to anyone—attempts to reach him may be as frustrating as attempting to undo the effects of abuse. These children often seem impervious to the efforts of teachers, counselors, and caregivers. Neither reward nor punishment seems to matter; the child appears to be equally unresponsive to both the giving and withholding of affection. Unfortunately, this has spanned a school of thought that promotes forcing children who suffer from "attachment disorders" into submission until they recognize their utter dependence on the parent or caregiver (DeAngelis, 1997).

Felix

After numerous moves through the homes of relatives and foster placements, 4-year-old Felix found a potential adoptive home with Connie. After a few weeks, Connie consulted a therapist because of her mounting frustration with Felix's misbehavior and refusal to follow her rules. The therapist diagnosed Felix as suffering from an attachment disorder and explained that unless Connie acted swiftly and forcefully, Felix would certainly grow up to be a monster with no control and no morals. He suggested a regimen of holding Felix until he could accept her love and nurturing. Connie followed the plan, which included holding a pillow over Felix's face when he fought against being cradled in her arms. The teachers at Felix's day care center began to worry about his growing agitation and fearfulness; when they asked him about bruises on his arms, he said that was where mommy had to hold him until he could learn to love her. They filed a report with Children's Protective Services. Following a psychiatric hospitalization, Felix was placed in a therapeutic foster home with a more benign approach to helping children form positive attachments.

The idea that children should be subjected to physical threats, violence, or verbal assaults and humiliation in order to force them into a relationship fails to consider the importance of the quality and nature of the relationship one hopes to create. We know too well that children who are abused form intense attachments to their abusers; despite broken bones and blackened eyes, they will insist upon the love they share with the parents who beat them. Using physical aggression to force a lost or frightened child into a relationship is easy; relying on love, tolerance and acceptance is far more difficult.

AFFECT REGULATION AND DISREGULATION

The child's capacity to regulate affect arises from interactions with the parent in the first months of life. The limbic system is essential in the origination of affect. Like other lower-brain structures, it only gradually comes under cortical control. Earlier investigators from the fields of sociology, anthropology, and psychology postulated the essential importance of mother–infant interaction on the infant's developing capacities for affect regulation as well as attachment behavior. More recent neurobiological research, which focuses on specific developmental changes in brain structure, supports the hypotheses generated from observational studies of primate and human infants. In his meticulous multidisciplinary review of research in these areas, Schore (1994) notes that discoveries of intense periods of myelination and synaptic growth in the limbic system and cortical areas of association correspond to critical periods in the development of attachment described by Bowlby (1973, 1980) and Mahler (1974). Thus, we see that the child is neurologically "primed" to absorb and organize specific kinds of experiences at varying points in early childhood (Emde & Buchsbaum, 1989).

The first 18 months of life are crucial for the neurobiological structuring of certain cortical pathways. These pathways allow an infant and child increasingly complex and sophisticated modulation of the affects and behavioral patterns that promote attachment to caregivers. Although the brain of the human infant is genetically predisposed to critical periods of synaptic proliferation and myelination, normative neurological development is absolutely dependent on "good enough" parenting (Winnicott, 1958), which allows for a multitude of characterologically and culturally determined variations in infant–caregiver interactions within an "average, expectable environment." Just as the infant, primed to develop language, will learn the language particular to his environment, the infant is primed for human interaction and will absorb the affects and ways of relating presented by his distinctive world.

The "loss of ability to regulate the intensity of feelings and impulses is possibly the most far-reaching effect of trauma and neglect" (van der Kolk & Fisler, 1994, p. 145). The behavior of children who have been abused is characterized by unpredictable impulsivity and inappropriately intense reactions to relatively subtle stimuli or a remarkable lack of response to even significant stimuli. Sometimes the frenzy is juxtaposed with a kind of psychic numbing that creates a somewhat bizarre shift between affective states. This can be understood as a diminution of or failure to achieve the ability to regulate affect, with a resulting decline in behavior that appears to the observer to be rationally motivated. Indeed, when stimuli, whether internally or externally generated, are not evaluated as to their place on a continuum from benign to life-threatening, the affective and behavioral responses they evoke are no longer under cortical control.

Ella

The child's loss of ability to modulate feelings was grimly demonstrated by Ella, who was referred to a therapeutic nursery school following the discovery that her father had repeatedly and brutally sexually assaulted her. After several months in the program, Ella had calmed considerably and had begun to relax with and trust her teachers and counselors. However, one day when her excited play was quickly moving toward uncontrolled frenzy, a trusted and familiar counselor quietly stepped toward her, intending to calmly sit with her until she regained control. As he moved to help her, Ella dropped to a crouch, as a look of terror crossed her face. The counselor asked Ella what she thought he was going to do. "Mess with my privates?" Ella responded.

Clearly, this interaction demonstrates far more than the disregulation of affect. However, it vividly shows the ways in which traumatized children can become frozen in a primitive world of intense and global affective responses. Over the course of childhood and adolescence, affective responses expand and become more nuanced. However, the affective repertoire of abused children is markedly diminished. Abuse sets in motion a neurological preparedness for an immediate response. The intense attentiveness to external stimuli associated with a "fight or flight" stance is mediated by catacholamines. There is now evidence that extended exposure to these alternations in catacholamine patterns may have a lasting effect on brainstem function (Gainotti & Caltagirone, 1989), such that the grossly overstimulated brain will always remain in a somewhat heightened state of readiness. Behaviorally, this means that a child may react more quickly or more intensely, to a perceived threat than we would expect, as did Ella.

Traumatized children essentially live in a chronic state of neurological "disregulation" (Perry, 1994). They behave almost as "emotional newborns" who may be described as living in an affectively binary world of either "distress or containment" (Krystal, 1988; Gazzaniga & LeDoux, 1978). To a child in this state, perceptions lack refinement. Actions and affects appear as global and undifferentiated entities; they are either dangerous or safe. In turn, the affective messages they send are equally generalized, often signaling only a readiness to fight or flee.

THE CREATION AND DISRUPTION OF MEMORY

Like affect regulation, memory appears to have its beginnings in the earliest infant–parent relationships and, initially, to involve the same areas of the brain. At first, processing of stimuli is highly context dependent; for example, the newborn shows special sensitivity to the smells, sounds, and touch of the caregiver. In particular, the visual cortex, which is highly developed at birth, is especially available for processing stimuli emanating from the external environment. Babies enjoy novel visual stimulation, particularly the gestalt of the human face.

In the earliest months of life, a baby can be passed from one smiling relative to another, happily responding to the different faces. When he encounters the familiar face of his mother, he may well show the excitement that comes with recognition. His behavior indicates to the observer that specific learning has taken place—that Mother's face has been stored in long-term memory. When an infant turns away from an unfamiliar face, we may assume that he has a memory of a particular face, against which he can compare the visual image before him. The new image may provide novelty and visual interest, or it may disturb him if he is searching for the face he associates with pleasure and comfort.

We recognize the infant's responsiveness to the sights, sounds, and smells of her caregiver as indicators, not only of her capacities for memory, but as a positive sign of attachment to them. When an infant or toddler shows evidence of indiscriminate responses to adults, we have cause for worry. This behavior indicates that the child's cognitive (and affective) memory of her caregiver is not associated with a sense of comfort, reassurance, or protection.

Two components of cognitive memory, recognition and recall, are sometimes considered as distinct processes or, alternatively, as aspects of a single, but multidimensional memory system (Noshpitz & King, 1991; Gazzaniga & LeDoux, 1978; Fair, 1992). Recognition describes the process by which a stimulus, whether originating internally or externally, is known as something familiar, even if not identical to a previously known stimulus. For example, on a walk through the park, we correctly classify Fido as a dog, even though we have never before encountered this particular animal.

Recall involves the bringing forth of information previously known but not presently in the conscious mind. At times this may be effortless and almost automatic, as when one picks up the phone and, without apparent thought, calls home. At other times, trying to retrieve a bit of information that one knows, but has forgotten, can be very difficult.

Memory relies on the reception, encoding, storage, and retrieval of information. The corpus callosum, the large fiber bundle that connects the left and right hemispheres of the brain, is essential for the distribution and retrieval of different aspects of received information, such as sensory impressions, meanings, or affective coloring, that comprise memory. The thalamus, hypothalamus, and the prefrontal cortex all participate in the processes of remembering and forgetting. The amygdala appears to be essential in the determination of which bits of information will go into long-term memory and is of special importance in the consideration of flashbacks. For example, when the amygdala is electrically stimulated during surgery, a patient experiences his memories as real—as occurring in the present, even when he knows that he is in surgery rather than in the kitchen of his childhood.

During the nervous system's response to abuse-induced trauma, the amygdala, along with other parts of subcortical areas, will be in a state of high excitation and at the same time bombarded with excessive, affectively laden stimuli. In this temporarily disabled state, the amygdala, along with other parts of the brain's memory system, may be unable to perform its usual functions. Therefore, information that would usually be subjected to examination before moving from perception to short-term to long-term memory, when received in an altered state of consciousness, may not undergo the usual neurological processes. Thus, these memories are stored as percepts, without the cortical processing of language, ordering, assessment, or assigning of meaning. Of equal importance, these are unwanted memories; there is a conscious wish to keep them out of the mind's eye.

We have all had the experience of being unable to recall something we consciously want to remember—the third item on the grocery list, the name of the person who just sat down next to us at a meeting or party, or the formula for solving the crucial problem on a final exam. Though these may seem important at the time, they are not lapses of recall about crucial events in our lives. Rather, they demonstrate minor lapses in cognitive or verbal memory. In instances like these, in order to "jar our memories," we may try to evoke visual or auditory clues as an aid to establishing a narrative context for the information that eludes us. Thus we say, "I was standing in front of the refrigerator when I realized we were out of . . . ," or "I can hear her voice, but I can't remember her name," or "If I could just see the first step of the formula, I know I'd remember the rest." So, when the verbal aspects of memory escape us, we turn to the episodic, pictorial representations of memory for assistance.

As described above, when a child's neurological response to the fear evoked by abuse is a hyperaroused stance, cortical activity is suppressed by the organism's sense of impending catastrophe. Consequently, what the child experiences in this state of consciousness will be remembered as fragmented sense impressions—images, feelings, or ideas disconnected from narrative structure. In contrast to our desire to recall the name of the person sitting next to us or the answer to an exam question, the child may have no wish to bring language to her memories of abuse. Because she does not wish to know what happened to her, she turns away from these fragments. Rather than using these episodic images to help her remember, she attempts to avoid the descriptive language, whether private or shared, that would reestablish the neuronal connections between the verbal, sensory, and affect-laden aspects of memory.

However, the powerful sights, sounds, and feelings of abuse are indelibly etched into the child's neuronal circuitry (Krystal, 1985; van der Kolk, Perry, & Herman, 1991). Because they are not stored in cortical or cognitive memory, they are not easily accessible by language-dependent recall, although they frequently show themselves in the child's play/actions and relationships/interactions. Unfortunately, they may also explode into the child's consciousness through flashbacks (Kaufman et al., 1997; Frankel, 1994), in which disparate pieces of an abusive event, or entire traumatic scenes, thrust themselves upon the unwary child's mind.

For most people, memories that come unbidden, whether a dream fragment called into consciousness by an unexpected visual image, or an intense feeling triggered by a seemingly forgotten smell, are not terrifying. Even if these remembrances are not pleasant, they are experienced as memories—an image or pattern of images from the past that has presented itself for consideration in the consciousness of the present. There is no loss of the "contemporaneous self." The person surprised by an unexpected memory is oriented to time, place, and person.

However, during a flashback, the person inundated by a traumatic memory may lose his orientation to time and place. This leaves him vulnerable to a retraumatization by memory; that is, because his experience is of living at the time and place of the traumatic event, all of the neurophysiological responses to the original trauma are reactivated. The original trauma has now been compounded.

Of course children's capacities to think, remember, and reason do not always involve abuse or flashbacks. It is often helpful to consider the disruptive effects of even relatively minor incidents in children's life experiences to remind us of the profound influences abuse can and does have. In the aftermath of a frightening experience, a child's memory for specific, verbally encoded memory may become inaccessible, leaving him vulnerable to the confusion and misapprehension that comes from not being able to remember correctly or think clearly.

Ben

For example, Ben loved dogs until a young but large German shepherd playfully pounced on him, knocking him to the ground. For the next several weeks, Ben screamed in terror at the sight of any unfamiliar

...itial profusely empathic response to Janie stemmed both from her
...nuine sympathy for this little girl and from her guilt over becoming
...noyed with Janie and seeing her as a clingy, whiny child. She had
...derstood Janie's hypervigilance and acute sensitivity to noises as a
...etition of the experiences with the cousin. During these episodes,
...ich occurred over a period of about 2 weeks, Janie and her cousin
...ld hide in the guest room. Not only did they have to be very quiet,
...they had to be very attentive to any noise, lest they be discovered.
...Janie's hypersensitivity to noise appeared to be the symptom most
...ptive to regular classroom activities. Her interruptions of morning
...e time" or quiet activities were so frequent that the class some-
...could not complete the activity. Initially the teacher had
...ed the usual protocol with Janie. She reminded Janie about not
...pting and then, if necessary, asked her to leave the circle until
...t able to maintain self-control. This obviously did not succeed.
...the therapist learned that the teacher had shifted to asking
...leave the room, she intervened.

...ether therapist and teacher decided on a plan for the times
...e most difficult for Janie: The assistant teacher would sit next
...ecidedly declining Janie's wish to sit in her lap, and either
...he noises or quietly remind her that the noises she was
...ere all "school noises." With the therapist's encouragement,
...rs became especially careful about explaining why any time
...the children to be quiet. These strategies seemed to have
...ct on Janie's behavior, yet their effect appeared to be
...t, leaving the teacher increasingly wondering if Janie's
...terruptions weren't a defiant bid for attention. After several
...ving Janie extra support, the teacher legitimately wanted
...to give more of her time to the other children in the
...rincipal echoed the teacher's concerns that they were
...rcing this "unwanted behavior."

...ultant wondered whether Janie's teacher might be more
...anie's hypervigilance and the resultant verbal disruptions
...d as symptoms, not only with meaning, but with a
...asis. With the consultant's help, the therapist came to
...possibility that Janie's hypervigilance and heightened
...might be both an indication of and result of the terror
...her cousin's assaults (Ornitz & Pynoos, 1989). As a
...uma, Janie had, at least temporarily, suffered a neuro-
...ased regression in her capacity to inhibit a panicked,

dog; he was only somewhat less frightened of dogs he knew and had previously liked. The leashed dog walking calmly on the opposite sidewalk evoked virtually the same response as the dog bounding toward him in the park. Ben was frightened but not physically hurt. Because he was not overwhelmingly terrified, Ben's fear of dogs faded relatively quickly by virtue of his parents' physical and verbal reassurances, his own retelling of his frightening experience, and repeated safe encounters with other dogs.

This vignette demonstrates the effects of Ben's temporary loss of the capacity to access specific memories of dogs. The affective association when he recognized a dog moved him into a state of hyperarousal that interfered with his capacity to evaluate his safety based on the available cues; he could not differentiate big dogs from little ones, mean ones from friendly ones.

These rudimentary sketches are intended to convey the complex interplay of internal and external factors in normal development and in potential neurophysiological responses to trauma. Although I have focused on the early months of life because of their critical importance in establishing the foundations for later development, common sense, as well as experience, tells us that, most fortunately, infantile experiences are not the sole determinants of personality, social behavior, or cognitive capacities. Later periods of intensive myelination and synaptic connections underlying the normative developmental crises of childhood, adolescence, and adulthood also allow for neurological and behavioral reorganizations.

Myelination and dendritic proliferation happen in predictable spurts throughout childhood, adolescence, and into early adulthood. Not surprisingly, critical periods of myelination, associated with cortical restructuring, are reflected in peak periods in the learning curve and/or major reorganizations in learning capabilities. Ornitz (1991) suggests that the four periods of major brain development, beginning with the neonatal period, followed by a spurt from ages 1 to 3, the third extending roughly from ages 6 to 10, and the spurt occurring during adolescence positively correlate with the shifts in Piagetian stages from sensorimotor, to preoperational to concrete operational, and formal operational learning (Inhelder & Piaget, 1958). The neurological development that continues into adulthood is characterized by consolidation of intracortical connections.

We can change our minds, and we can change our brains—within limits. Brain cells that are damaged or destroyed do not regenerate, but new pathways can be found. Psychotherapy aims to repair, restore, or initiate neurological processes that have been damaged, rendered inoperable, or were never created because of the traumatic effects of abuse.

At any moment, millions of discrete pieces of information impinge on our central nervous system; nerve cells are in a state of continual activity, simultaneously exciting and inhibiting each other in the reception, sorting, discarding, storing, and retrieval of massive amounts of information around and within us. When the system works well, we continually make conscious and unconscious choices about how and where to direct our attention. For example, we might concentrate on discreet information in the process of learning or allow our minds to wander until an internal or external snippet captures our attention. When this system is disrupted, thinking, learning, and memory become exceedingly difficult. For children who have been abused, these activities may actually become impossible, at least some of the time, because of the disturbance in normal neurological processes. We cannot directly view the distortions in brain function that come from abuse, but we can see them only too clearly when pathological thinking or behavior intrudes.

Abusive experiences disrupt neurophysiological foundations of attachment, memory, and the regulation of affect. From these traumas arise the patterns of pathological behavior characteristic of abused children. However, the meanings of the shared symptoms are unique to each child and dependent on the personal experience and history that precede and follow the abuse.

The child's capacity to symbolize and bring language to memories of abuse potentially allows for integration and recovery (van der Kolk & Fisler, 1994). It is not only the conscious making of meaning that is curative but the effects that talking produces on the neuronal communication between different functional centers of the brain. As nonverbal memories gradually become accessible to and ordered by language, the child's vulnerability to intrusions of overwhelming affect diminishes, and her capacity to tolerate the intimacy of human relationships increases. Thus, the recovery from abuse can best be aided if one remains cognizant of the complex interplay of mind and brain.

As the following vignette demonstrates, the clinician who appreciates the physiological, as well as psychological, consequences of

abuse can then educate others about the patience req recovers. During this period, the child may need pr unrealistic expectations and demands of those recuperate more quickly than is possible.

Janie

Janie had always required a great deal of adul she demanded almost constant care from her complained of vague somatic symptoms whe much time with her as she wished. Janie learned that a visiting adolescent cousin h episodes of "doctor" play, involving mutual masturbating to orgasm while Janie watch with her cousin, Janie's somatic compla awareness of the smallest scrape, bump, bodies of her teacher and classmates. In pected noise startled her. Her freque "What's wrong?", "Where'd that sound to take their toll in the classroom.

At the request of her mother consulted with school personnel sho ning of therapy. Over the next seve conversations with the teacher, w been extremely sympathetic and s somatic complaints and const teacher's mounting irritation.

The therapist found herself partly in response to the teach about the ineffectiveness of that the teacher's anger to empathy, she struggled agair had to control herself." F approach but the meaning and the teacher, the ther

The consultant was sophisticated psychologi in relation to her perso Janie and her teacher.

global response to unexpected noises. In addition, rather than accommodating herself to repeated unexpected sounds, that is, having responses gradually diminishing in intensity, Janie's hyperarousal made her tend in the other direction. So, for example, while the other children in her class may have initially noticed a loud or unusual noise but become gradually less responsive to it as it repeated, Janie became increasingly sensitive to these surprising sounds. In essence, in a state of alertness, the other children could accurately assess the situation and, having realized that they were not in danger, return to the task at hand. However, Janie rapidly moved into a state of hyperarousal in which she could not make an accurate assessment of her situation. Rather than adapting to unexpected noises, Janie, in effect, became retraumatized with every new and unusual auditory experience. Naturally, therefore, the mechanics of reading or arithmetic were eluding her, and she was constantly seeking attention and reassurance.

The teacher had responded instinctively to Janie's regressed behavior with the offer of added support; if Janie's symptoms had stemmed from one of the many minor and expectable setbacks of childhood, such as an illness, a parent's unexpected or extended absence, or the birth of a sibling, a few days or weeks of extra attention would likely have enabled Janie to get back on track. However, along with all of the complex feelings bombarding Janie during her cousin's sexual assaults, her intense fear resulted in neurological changes. Previously reliable neuronal pathways had been overwhelmed during the abuse and continued to remain inaccessible to Janie. Until they were restored to their previous level of functional maturity, Janie would quite literally be physically unable to remain calm in the classroom. Expecting her to do so would be as fruitless as expecting a dyslexic child simply to stop perceiving letters as reversed!

A thorough consideration of this particular symptom allowed the therapist to realize that she had probably underestimated the extent of Janie's fear during the incidents with her cousin. With heightened appreciation for how truly overwhelmed Janie had felt and continued to feel, the therapist could now approach Janie's teacher with a more complete explanation for the apparent intractability of Janie's regressive fears and demands. While the teacher had recognized Janie's need for additional support, neither she, the therapist, nor Janie's parents had fully grasped the enormity of the tasks facing Janie. The resources to meet Janie's needs simply were not available within the classroom.

Janie's parents had been understandably reluctant to do anything that would violate her privacy. They felt that Janie's privacy had already been disregarded, not only by the abusive cousin, but by the physical exam and interviews that followed her disclosure. This position had argued against their doing anything at school to call special attention to Janie. However, they could now see that Janie's behavior had already made her the focus of considerable negative attention from teachers and peers alike. Since Janie's symptoms had not abated as quickly as they had originally hoped, they readily agreed to the therapist's proposal that a full-time volunteer, whose primary responsibility would be to assist Janie, be assigned to Janie's classroom. Although her primary focus would be to help Janie cope with the many previously manageable, but now overwhelming, demands of classroom life, the aide would also be available to help the teacher and the other children as needs arose. The expectation was that as Janie's capacities for affect regulation improved, she would require less and less individual attention and could be helped to reintegrate herself into the group.

When the teacher understood that, like a learning disability, Janie's symptomatic behavior had an organic basis, she became intrigued with developing strategies to help Janie cope with this interference in her capacity to learn. Previously she had noted that Janie's work had become exceedingly disorganized. She now considered the possibility that Janie quite literally could not order her thoughts or effectively organize her written work. The therapist agreed that her earlier explanation that the messiness of Janie's work reflected her internal state of disarray, while true, was incomplete. She was excited by the teacher's proposal to approach some of Janie's difficulties as she would a child with definable problems in sequencing and spatial planning. Previously the teacher had felt that her role with Janie was essentially passive, that is, that, other than offering comfort and reassurance, her task was really to wait until Janie and her therapist resolved the psychological issues so that Janie could begin to learn again. She now saw herself as having an active role in helping Janie learn to cope with and master her symptoms. Consequently, she began to offer strategies to help diminish Janie's disorganization, for example, by giving her the materials for an art project in several small, manageable amounts, rather than all at once. As Janie could organize both more and increasingly complex stimuli, the teacher could adjust her expectations accordingly.

The recognition of the sources of Janie's regressed cognitive state allowed the teacher comfortably to lower her expectations for Janie without feeling that she was either "giving in to" or encouraging regression. Clearly circle time was impossible for Janie; even with constant adult attention—she simply could not process all of the stimulation that this activity produced. Her fearfulness and disorganized behavior reflected her nervous system's temporary inability to inhibit irrelevant stimuli and effectively order relevant information.

Consequently, instead of joining the group, Janie and the aide left the room to go on a "sound search" throughout the school. Initially, Janie was very frightened, often more so when things were too quiet than when they were very noisy, clinging to the aide for comfort and reassurance. The aide encouraged Janie's tentative explorations but allowed Janie to titrate gradual moves toward independent activity. After a few weeks Janie could comfortably move about the school without requiring an adult in immediate proximity. As expected, the "sound search" began to seem babyish and boring. When Janie protested leaving the room at circle time, she was invited back into the group. (The teacher had wisely acquiesced to other children's requests to go on "sound searches," thereby helping to keep Janie integrated into the class while temporarily offering her a special curriculum.)

Fortunately, as is sometimes the case, particularly where language is concerned, strategies initially designed to manage symptoms can actually help reduce the problem underlying the symptoms. For example, to help Janie become desensitized to the cacophony of sounds permeating her elementary school, with consultation from the therapist, the teacher and the new aide developed several games for Janie involving auditory discrimination. The exercises focused on identifying the sources of different sounds, naming affects associated with noises, and distinguishing between quiet and loud sounds. In helping Janie bring language to frightening sensory experiences, these activities were actually enabling Janie to establish neuronal pathways to replace those that had apparently been rendered useless by her neurochemical response to a situation in which she felt overwhelming terror. In turn, as Janie regained her previous capacity for language, she could begin to put words to an experience that apparently had been taken in and stored as nameless fragments of sight and sound. In essence, the more language she had to use, the more Janie could use language, which, in turn, gave her more language to use.

As she came to see herself as an active participant in Janie's recovery, the teacher's impatience began to diminish. This allayed the therapist's sense of responsibility for "curing" Janie in order to avoid the teacher's disapproval. Before she had felt both internal and external pressure to teach Janie to behave. She now felt in a position to help Janie learn about herself; when Janie became terrified of an unexpected noise during a therapy session, the therapist could attend to the immediate affect and Janie's sense of helplessness. She began to talk with Janie about how unhappy she felt when she couldn't make her body hold still or when her thoughts went so fast she couldn't stop them. Together Janie and her therapist could explore how upsetting it was for Janie to feel so unable to control her own body, not only in the face of the unexpected and unwanted assaults from her cousin, but from the internal intrusions of unexpected and unwanted images and affects.

In this case, resources were available to create a milieu in which educational and therapeutic approaches could be integrated in a mutually supportive manner. However, in order to develop an integrated approach to treatment, no matter how limited or grand the resources, one must have a diagnostic assessment that recognizes the complex interplay of the emotional and cognitive, social and individual, and psychological and physiological factors.

We come to know the mind of another through our interpersonal affective and behavioral exchanges. But perhaps we do not often stop to consider that it is through this process that we come to know something about the workings of the brain of another. In this regard, I think of the many times I listen to a story of a disrupted, neglectful, or abusive childhood and wonder how the person sitting before me could possibly be as psychologically healthy as he appears to be. As the story unfolds, I am not surprised to find that somewhere in the midst of all of the upset and psychological turmoil there was an important, nurturing, life-sustaining relationship. From a psychoanalytic perspective, we are used to thinking that the relationship may well have saved the child from insanity. From the above, it should also be clear that this relationship may also have spared the child serious brain damage.

It is crucial to recognize that one can neither damage nor protect the child's mind without equally influencing the brain in either direction. We undertake psychotherapy with children who have been abused in an attempt to minimize the ongoing harm to their psyches and brains. We must simultaneously know that both the mind and the brain are resilient and that recovery always exacts a price. Children who have been hurt can learn to love, trust, remember without fear, and monitor their affective responses. With our help, previously functional neurological processes can be restored or new, more reliable mechanisms can be created, but we cannot remove the facts of abuse from the child's brain or mind.

Chapter Five

Memory and Disclosure

Some children readily tell us the facts of abuse, and some do so reluctantly; others endure emotional, physical, or sexual assault for months or even years without deliberately and clearly articulating their plight to someone in a position to help. Though these children sometimes feel that they tried to tell someone, or that the grown-ups around them should have known that something was wrong, they often cannot identify, even as adults, precisely what prevented them from clearly voicing their troubles.

Obviously, children do not talk about every event in their lives with parents, teachers, or friends. Nor do they ask for clarification every time they feel confused. We should therefore make certain to consider not only *whether* children tell us when they feel in danger or have been hurt, but *how* they inform us about both inconsequential and important events, ideas, and feelings and *what* they choose or are able to divulge.

Even those with no knowledge of psychoanalytic theory intuitively sense the complications of remembering and forgetting. We intentionally search our memories for maddeningly elusive informa-

I am indebted to Jane Hewitt, my late classmate, colleague, and friend, for her typically unabashed and cogent remarks on this chapter. As was her wont, she pushed me to clarify my thoughts—in this instance about why some children talk about abuse and others do not.

tion yet are plagued by the memory of a melody or scene that seems almost deliberate in its refusal to leave us in peace. Because of its historical emphasis on transference, as well as the verbal reconstruction of childhood events and relationships, psychoanalytic investigation has ceded a pivotal place to memory, both in general considerations of theory and the particulars of individual therapy.

When the criminal prosecution of an alleged perpetrator of abuse or the attempt to gain financial compensation for physical or emotional injury rests on a child's memory, those involved in the investigations may have both a different attitude toward and a different purpose for understanding children's capacities and incapacities for accurate memory. Just as it behooves any therapist treating abused children to know something about the neurological underpinnings of trauma-induced symptoms, the therapist will be well served, not only in his direct work with children, but also in his contacts with social workers, investigators, and attorneys, to understand the cognitive and psychological underpinnings of memory.

In general, children demonstrate little evidence of memory for events in the first 3 years of life. They lack both the neural structure for encoding and active retrieval as well as the linguistic capacities essential for creating narrative structure (Tessler & Nelson, 1996). Like traumatic memories, events experienced preverbally do not easily find verbal expression, although Hewitt (1994) reports on psychotherapy with two little girls whose preverbal behavior suggested unconfirmed sexual abuse. When these children developed sufficient language, they described, primitively though powerfully, the molestation for which they earlier had no words.

Multiple factors influence the strength, organization, and content of children's memories. Information that resembles previously acquired knowledge is more easily remembered than something entirely new. Because of this, a teacher may present multiplication by demonstrating the characteristics it shares with addition. Many months or years later the children, having memorized their multiplication tables, may have little memory of the experience of first learning them. However, if an unusual and emotionally charged event occurred during the learning experience—an earthquake, a tornado striking, the teacher's fainting, or an errant puppy wandering into the classroom—they would be more likely to recall that specific lesson because of the affective charge associated with it. To a large extent, children's memories of events are socially constructed (Tessler & Nelson, 1996) through an interactive dog; he was only somewhat less frightened of dogs he knew and had previously liked. The leashed dog walking calmly on the opposite sidewalk evoked virtually the same response as the dog bounding toward him in the park. Ben was frightened but not physically hurt. Because he was not overwhelmingly terrified, Ben's fear of dogs faded relatively quickly by virtue of his parents' physical and verbal reassurances, his own retelling of his frightening experience, and repeated safe encounters with other dogs.

This vignette demonstrates the effects of Ben's temporary loss of the capacity to access specific memories of dogs. The affective association when he recognized a dog moved him into a state of hyperarousal that interfered with his capacity to evaluate his safety based on the available cues; he could not differentiate big dogs from little ones, mean ones from friendly ones.

These rudimentary sketches are intended to convey the complex interplay of internal and external factors in normal development and in potential neurophysiological responses to trauma. Although I have focused on the early months of life because of their critical importance in establishing the foundations for later development, common sense, as well as experience, tells us that, most fortunately, infantile experiences are not the sole determinants of personality, social behavior, or cognitive capacities. Later periods of intensive myelination and synaptic connections underlying the normative developmental crises of childhood, adolescence, and adulthood also allow for neurological and behavioral reorganizations.

Myelination and dendritic proliferation happen in predictable spurts throughout childhood, adolescence, and into early adulthood. Not surprisingly, critical periods of myelination, associated with cortical restructuring, are reflected in peak periods in the learning curve and/or major reorganizations in learning capabilities. Ornitz (1991) suggests that the four periods of major brain development, beginning with the neonatal period, followed by a spurt from ages 1 to 3, the third extending roughly from ages 6 to 10, and the spurt occurring during adolescence positively correlate with the shifts in Piagetian stages from sensorimotor, to preoperational to concrete operational, and formal operational learning (Inhelder & Piaget, 1958). The neurological development that continues into adulthood is characterized by consolidation of intracortical connections.

We can change our minds, and we can change our brains—within limits. Brain cells that are damaged or destroyed do not regenerate, but new pathways can be found. Psychotherapy aims to repair, restore, or initiate neurological processes that have been damaged, rendered inoperable, or were never created because of the traumatic effects of abuse.

At any moment, millions of discrete pieces of information impinge on our central nervous system; nerve cells are in a state of continual activity, simultaneously exciting and inhibiting each other in the reception, sorting, discarding, storing, and retrieval of massive amounts of information around and within us. When the system works well, we continually make conscious and unconscious choices about how and where to direct our attention. For example, we might concentrate on discreet information in the process of learning or allow our minds to wander until an internal or external snippet captures our attention. When this system is disrupted, thinking, learning, and memory become exceedingly difficult. For children who have been abused, these activities may actually become impossible, at least some of the time, because of the disturbance in normal neurological processes. We cannot directly view the distortions in brain function that come from abuse, but we can see them only too clearly when pathological thinking or behavior intrudes.

Abusive experiences disrupt neurophysiological foundations of attachment, memory, and the regulation of affect. From these traumas arise the patterns of pathological behavior characteristic of abused children. However, the meanings of the shared symptoms are unique to each child and dependent on the personal experience and history that precede and follow the abuse.

The child's capacity to symbolize and bring language to memories of abuse potentially allows for integration and recovery (van der Kolk & Fisler, 1994). It is not only the conscious making of meaning that is curative but the effects that talking produces on the neuronal communication between different functional centers of the brain. As nonverbal memories gradually become accessible to and ordered by language, the child's vulnerability to intrusions of overwhelming affect diminishes, and her capacity to tolerate the intimacy of human relationships increases. Thus, the recovery from abuse can best be aided if one remains cognizant of the complex interplay of mind and brain.

As the following vignette demonstrates, the clinician who appreciates the physiological, as well as psychological, consequences of abuse can then educate others about the patience required as the child recovers. During this period, the child may need protection from the unrealistic expectations and demands of those who want her to recuperate more quickly than is possible.

Janie

Janie had always required a great deal of adult attention. At school she demanded almost constant care from her teachers and frequently complained of vague somatic symptoms when they couldn't spend as much time with her as she wished. Janie was 6 when her parents learned that a visiting adolescent cousin had engaged her in several episodes of "doctor" play, involving mutual genital exploration and his masturbating to orgasm while Janie watched. Following the episodes with her cousin, Janie's somatic complaints intensified, as did her awareness of the smallest scrape, bump, or bruise on her body and the bodies of her teacher and classmates. In addition, the slightest unexpected noise startled her. Her frequent questions—"What's that?", "What's wrong?", "Where'd that sound come from?"—were beginning to take their toll in the classroom.

At the request of her mother and teacher, Janie's therapist had consulted with school personnel shortly after the abuse, at the beginning of therapy. Over the next several weeks she also had many phone conversations with the teacher, whose initial response to Janie had been extremely sympathetic and solicitous. However, Janie's unceasing somatic complaints and constant disruptive questions fueled the teacher's mounting irritation.

The therapist found herself growing equally impatient with Janie, partly in response to the teacher's annoyance and quiet implications about the ineffectiveness of treatment. As the therapist recognized that the teacher's anger toward Janie was quickly surpassing her empathy, she struggled against the impulse to tell Janie that she "just had to control herself." Recognizing not only the futility of this approach but the meanings it had for her relationship with both Janie and the teacher, the therapist sought consultation.

The consultant was impressed with the therapist's thorough and sophisticated psychological analysis of Janie's symptoms, their meaning in relation to her personality structure, and the relationship between Janie and her teacher. The therapist had recognized that the teacher's initial profusely empathic response to Janie stemmed both from her genuine sympathy for this little girl and from her guilt over becoming annoyed with Janie and seeing her as a clingy, whiny child. She had understood Janie's hypervigilance and acute sensitivity to noises as a repetition of the experiences with the cousin. During these episodes, which occurred over a period of about 2 weeks, Janie and her cousin would hide in the guest room. Not only did they have to be very quiet, but they had to be very attentive to any noise, lest they be discovered.

Janie's hypersensitivity to noise appeared to be the symptom most disruptive to regular classroom activities. Her interruptions of morning "circle time" or quiet activities were so frequent that the class sometimes could not complete the activity. Initially the teacher had followed the usual protocol with Janie. She reminded Janie about not interrupting and then, if necessary, asked her to leave the circle until she felt able to maintain self-control. This obviously did not succeed. When the therapist learned that the teacher had shifted to asking Janie to leave the room, she intervened.

Together therapist and teacher decided on a plan for the times that were most difficult for Janie: The assistant teacher would sit next to her, decidedly declining Janie's wish to sit in her lap, and either identify the noises or quietly remind her that the noises she was hearing were all "school noises." With the therapist's encouragement, the teachers became especially careful about explaining *why* any time they asked the children to be quiet. These strategies seemed to have some impact on Janie's behavior, yet their effect appeared to be intermittent, leaving the teacher increasingly wondering if Janie's constant interruptions weren't a defiant bid for attention. After several weeks of giving Janie extra support, the teacher legitimately wanted her assistant to give more of her time to the other children in the class. The principal echoed the teacher's concerns that they were merely reinforcing this "unwanted behavior."

The consultant wondered whether Janie's teacher might be more responsive if Janie's hypervigilance and the resultant verbal disruptions were presented as symptoms, not only with meaning, but with a neurological basis. With the consultant's help, the therapist came to appreciate the possibility that Janie's hypervigilance and heightened startle response might be both an indication of and result of the terror Janie felt during her cousin's assaults (Ornitz & Pynoos, 1989). As a result of this trauma, Janie had, at least temporarily, suffered a neurophysiologically based regression in her capacity to inhibit a panicked, through this dangerous territory safely yet again. In contrast to his fearfulness, Paul's parents were apparently oblivious to the dangers to which they regularly subjected themselves and their children; they drove and chatted in the front seat as if nothing were wrong.

I asked what he was afraid of: "The Korean War." He explained with a chuckle that he had been "absolutely convinced that the Korean War was being fought on the roof of that barn." He did not recall how his fear gradually faded away or what caused him, many years later, to remember those scary rides. He also didn't know for sure why he had never told his parents until, a few months earlier, he had mentioned his terrifying scenario to his mother. This was the first she had heard of Paul's baffling childhood fear.

Jared

Jared, a boy of about 12, one day mused to his mother, "Do you remember when you took me and Sam [his best friend] to Dr. Stone's to get those shots?" His mother, searching her memory, replied, "I've never taken you and Sam to Dr. Stone's." "Yes, you did," he continued. "Don't you remember? And Sam's mother went with us."

Jared's mother was curious about this conversation, since these events, about which he seemed to have such a clear memory, were so unlikely to have occurred. The next time she saw Sam's mother, she asked whether her friend recalled this event. Her friend was equally baffled by Jared's recollection.

Alice

Alice, a successful professional woman in her 40s, told me the following story. As a young adolescent, she had spent a summer working in the family business. Shortly after she began her summer job, she told her mother that one of the long-time employees was making her quite uncomfortable. Initially she wondered if his standing too close or seeming to brush against her or touch her unnecessarily as they passed in the hall was just her imagination. When, on one occasion, she felt he quite clearly and deliberately touched her breast, Alice went to her mother.

She remembered that her mother responded calmly, expressed regret that this had happened, and thanked her for telling her what was going on. She assured Alice that nothing like it would ever happen again. To the best of her knowledge, that was the end of it.

Alice had no memory of any further discussions with either of her parents. The employee resumed his previous friendly and respectful relationship with her and continued to work in the family business until his retirement many years later.

The first two examples concern external events that didn't actually happen. The Korean War was not fought on American soil, and Jared did not go to Dr. Stone's as part of a foursome. Instead, they illustrate children's use of the external world to manage internal experiences.

When Paul told his story, he was not relaying a memory of the Korean War being fought in the farmlands of the American midwest but, rather, his memory of a childhood experience of being afraid and confused by an idea that he had created from bits and pieces of internal and external reality then externalized in the form of a frightening image. Though as an adult he was rather amused by his creation, his correction of his childhood distortion still leaves unanswered questions.

Which elements of his internal experiences became absorbed into his understanding of world events such that a conflict thousands of miles away was moved virtually into his backyard? Did this successfully, even if temporarily, solve a dilemma for him? Perhaps, for example, by confining this intense battle to the roof of a barn, he felt freer from conflict when he was away from the barn. But, in the context of the present discussion, we must wonder why he didn't mention his fears to his parents.

In the case of Jared, by talking more with him about the details of his memory, his mother was able to understand Jared's account. At his 6-year annual exam, Dr. Stone had told Jared that he would not have to have any more immunizations until he was a teenager. Since he was somewhat frightened of injections, Jared was thrilled. His mother remembered his almost tearful relief at this announcement.

Two years later, during his annual exam, Dr. Stone unexpectedly announced that a new vaccine had become available that he was recommending for all of his patients. Despite Jared's tearful protests, his mother and Dr. Stone agreed that he should have the vaccine. The injection was administered, and he left the pediatrician's office furious that Dr. Stone had broken his promise.

In reality, this had been a very upsetting experience for Jared. He had been caught off-guard and humiliated by the intensity of his feelings. He had also felt betrayed by two trusted adults. His memory had transformed this experience into a more palatable scenario.

In the revised version, Jared and his best friend went together to the pediatrician for the express purpose of getting the new vaccine. He was neither surprised nor alone. He was also able to titrate his rage at and disappointment in his mother by including Sam's mother among the culprits; this became something many parents had done to their children, rather than a particular injury his mother had inflicted on him. Interestingly, Jared had neither repressed the memory, "forgotten" the experience, nor created a scenario in which he escaped the dreaded injection. Thus, the particular distortions of Jared's memory make it clear that it was the feelings about himself and those he relied upon to care for him, not the physical pain of the injection, that were so intolerable that they necessitated an historical revision.

If we were to talk to all of the children in Dr. Stone's practice who were told they were finished with immunizations and later informed that they had to endure another injection, we would undoubtedly hear a variety of stories. For many, the memory of the event would probably pretty closely match the "historical truth." For others, the memory might be vague or inaccessible; and still others, like Jared, might have created a memory that made the internalization of an unpleasant experience easier.

Why did Jared mention this memory to his mother? "Because it seemed kind of funny." Jared was aware that this memory was not consistent with his experience; something didn't quite fit. In asking his mother about it, he was attempting to come to terms with the unsettled feeling the memory engendered.

We want children to ask us about events, feelings, and ideas that "seem kind of funny." We want to know about the things that make them uncomfortable, frightened, or hurt. By talking to his mother, Jared was able to clarify a relatively inconsequential event in his childhood. However, this memory may still undergo many modifications over the course of childhood and adolescence. It is not clear what importance it may have or in what form it may be stored. Because Jared wanted to discuss the memory with his mother, it is unlikely that he will store it in the form he presented to her. It might be revised to match more closely the events as they occurred. Alternatively, deprived of its affective charge, it might fade. Jared supplanted the original unsettling experience with a distorted memory, which, though more affectively acceptable, created an unsettling cognitive dissonance. Since the conversation gave both Jared and his mother the opportunity to clarify the distortions and rework the fear and hurt feelings, the memory of the conversation itself might become the most prominent aspect of this series of events and memories.

This appears to be the case concerning Alice's memory of the incipient sexual molestation. Alice's clearest memory of the discrete events involved in this incident was of talking with her mother. Alice was able to rely, not only on the interpersonal relationship with her mother for help and comfort, but on the intrapsychic representation of her mother as a consoling, protective figure. Obviously, the mother had not been able to prevent the initial sexual advances, but the demonstration of her power to influence Alice's environment was sufficient that Alice was able to retain the incident in conscious memory without undue anxiety and, as an adult, feel that this incident was a relatively minor negative experience that had little effect on her life.

So if Jared approached his parent about a memory that seemed to him to be "not quite right" and Alice approached her parent about an incident that made her distinctly uncomfortable, why did Paul sit through months of terror without broaching his fears with his parents? Possibly his silence stemmed from the incongruity he sensed between his feelings and his parents' behavior. After all, while he was quivering with fear in the back seat, they were in the front seat behaving as if nothing were amiss, as if there were no Korean War on the barn roof. Perhaps their behavior introduced some doubt into his conviction about the veracity of his ideas, which, in turn, may have created a sense of tension, conscious or not, about whether his fears stemmed from a real or imagined danger. Yet, if we suppose that at some point Paul, again possibly not entirely consciously, assumed that the proximity of the Korean War to his home was a product of his imagination, we may still wonder why he did not present it to his parents as just that. Children do, after all, recognize that their understandings of the world are altered by emotional and intellectual growth. They often proudly and eagerly announce what they "used to" think, or remind themselves and their parents of past fears that have come to seem silly or infantile.

However, to make such a declaration requires the child consciously to feel the belief sufficiently "historical" that he will not be embarrassed by having it known. If a child "knows" intellectually that he should not be afraid yet continues to feel frightened, he is vulnerable to feeling diminished in his own eyes as well as in his parents' estimation of him. Perhaps for this child, the tension between reality and fantasy was not sufficiently resolved for him to raise the question to his parents. What if his beliefs weren't true, as their behavior suggested? Would they be angry, would they laugh at his foolishness, or not believe him? What if he were right? Would they be angry that he had not spoken up earlier, had not tried to protect them from danger? Perhaps Paul concluded that it would be better just to say nothing at all rather than risk the consequences of speaking one's mind.

By and large, children probably do not tell parents the ideas and feelings they feel will too greatly disturb their images of themselves, their parents, and the parent–child relationship. If children believe that disclosure of abuse will diminish them in their parents' eyes, not only because they fear a parent's anger or punishment for crimes of thought or action, but also because they believe the parent will think poorly of them, they are less likely to reveal their thoughts. When a child expects that an affective communication will receive an emotional response, similar both in kind and in intensity, he or she can freely talk to a parent, teacher, or therapist. The expectation is more than an assumption that the adult will see the child's point of view; it rests on the often unarticulated belief that the adult will respond empathically to the child's feelings and will adapt his or her emotional response to meet the child's needs.

When children expect that adults will not be attuned to them, they frequently do not talk about the very things with which they need the most help. For example, it is not uncommon to hear that a child did not inform her parent about childhood abuse because she expected that the parent would be "too upset" or that it would cause "too much trouble" in the extended family or with friendships. Even when the child anticipates the appropriate parental responses of anger, sadness, or horror at what had happened to her, if she nevertheless feels that these reactions would differ from her own affective experience, for example, in their intensity, she may not go to them for help. In these cases, the child may fear destroying the relationship to the internalized parent. From a young age, a child relies on internal images of parents for comfort, guidance, support, and discipline, measuring herself and her behavior against her sense of her parents' expectations of her and their relationship. If she believes that a disclosure of abuse will irreparably disrupt or overwhelm a tenuously structured relationship, she is likely to keep quiet in order to preserve the relationship. This may happen without conscious thought, just as a child may avoid taking her concerns to a parent who seems to be or she feels *is* too fragile to bear them.

However, it is important to remember that children do not always correctly read adult responses and that their expectations and interpretations are subject to distortions based on their own emotional processes. For example, one frequently hears from adults that they grew up without any discussions with their parents about sex. The typical explanation for this lapse is the parents' embarrassment or discomfort. Of course, this may be entirely true, but it omits the possibility that the child's embarrassment may have contributed equally to the apparent lack of sex education.

After all, children do often experience their sexual curiosity as illicit, expecting to be chastised or punished for wanting to know about something that they understand is part of private adult relationships. So while children may complain that their parents never talked to them about sex, parents are often amused or baffled when their attempts to talk with their children about sex are met with an embarrassed silence, a quick reassurance that sex education at school "took care of all of that," or the child's sudden realization that a long overdue library book has to be returned at the very moment his father wants to talk about sex! In some instances both parents and children may remember these interactions; in other cases the child may entirely forget that such an affectively charged exchange ever took place.

Children may both forget or become confused about what they have been told by adults and what they have said to adults. Consider the mundane examples that repeatedly occur in the daily lives of families. As she is about to walk out the door for school, Lauren wails, "I don't have the notebook I need for science." Mother replies, "What notebook? Do you need a new one?" "I told you I did. You never listen to me!" Something was forgotten here. Did Lauren forget that she *didn't* tell her mother or did her mother forget that she *did*?

Exchanges like these remind us of the murkiness that can surround the exchange of information about relatively inconsequential as well as important matters. When considering children's remembered attempts to inform parents or other adults about physical or sexual abuse, we must not forget that children sometimes overestimate their efforts to let someone know what is on their minds. When Lauren protests, "I told you, but you never listen!" she conveys her frustration at her needs not being met. If indeed she does repeatedly tell her mother what she needs and her mother *doesn't* listen, Lauren will rightly feel a sense of helplessness and isolation. Alternatively, if Lauren merely intended to speak up about what she needed, or if she approached her mother about the science notebook when her mother was distracted, then we might view Lauren's sense of helpless frustration somewhat differently. If we unquestioningly accept a child's "I told them, but they didn't listen," we may inadvertently shore up a sense of helplessness and isolation unsupported by external reality.

A child's wish to speak clearly and directly may color her sense of having done so, particularly if she is uncertain about whether what she has to say is "true," or isn't really sure what words to use, or what, exactly she is afraid of. When a child feels that she has spoken unambiguously but not been heard, or that the import of her message was ignored, her sense of outrage at an insensitive listener would be justified. She might also feel enormously sad and alone, with little hope that adults would offer the care or protection she so urgently needs.

On the other hand, if her efforts to tell her story have been muted or have occurred largely through well-disguised "hints," it will be helpful for her to understand what contributed to her being less clear than she might have been. Such an understanding will ultimately diminish her sense of aloneness and provide opportunities for her to become more effective in getting what she needs from adults.

Unfortunately, a very dangerous paradox lurks here. Children should *not* be in the business of reporting sexual or physical abuse. For children in this miserable position—of having to explain to one or several adults that they have been physically, sexually, or emotionally abused—the world has gone terribly, terribly wrong.

Children are entitled to protection from abuse. When we, as individuals or a community, fail to keep them safe, we must accept full responsibility for the harm that has befallen them. This seems very simple, yet when we turn our attention away from this notion and begin educating abused children about "good touch and bad touch" or start trying to teach them about how to speak up in their own behalf, we send a very clear message that they bear at least partial responsibility for the injuries they have suffered—and this is decidedly *not* therapeutic. We must learn to say to children, both implicitly and explicitly, "I should not have let that happen to you!" instead of "Why didn't you tell me?"

Understandably, but all too often, abused children feel that they cannot rely on adults to care for them. When we set out to teach them how to care for themselves, should danger appear again, we support their view that they are and should have been responsible for their own care. This is a bit like greeting someone whose home has been destroyed by arson with instructions on the proper installation of smoke alarms. It suggests that the problem lay in the failure of a warning system rather than with the arsonist who caused the blaze.

The pernicious effects of this message cannot be overstated. Abused children do not easily turn to adults for aid and comfort; dependence on another does not come readily. This is where we need to direct our attention, rather than to increasing their self-help skills.

I do not mean to suggest that we abandon all efforts to help children protect themselves; I do want to stress that we must not covertly blame them when they, for whatever reason, could not call for help. Our efforts may involve helping these children to confront the realities of living in an impossible environment—one in which the adults responsible for their care could not or did not protect them. For abused children and their therapists, this may pose a very difficult task. If the therapist's explicit messages are directed toward absolving the child of her unwarranted guilt by blaming the parent, while the child's efforts are toward protecting the parent, their attempts to communicate will surely fail. The child will again feel betrayed and misunderstood.

Assisting a child in understanding all of the factors that made it difficult or impossible for her to get help when she needed it will be therapeutic if, and only if, the child comes to absolve herself of responsibility. We will certainly have to help her struggle with the complicated feelings, perceptions, misperceptions, ideas, and relationships that made it difficult or impossible for her to get help. In many cases this requires a very delicate touch in helping the child understand her motivations and behavior without appearing to either condone or blame.

Cora

After Cora's parents divorced, her father would often come into her bed when she spent weekends with him. She would feign sleep as he predictably first stroked her legs and stomach before fondling her vulva and inserting his fingers into her vagina. At the age of 11, she knew this was wrong of him; it make her almost sick to think about what was happening, but when she didn't really think about it, it felt good. She also desperately loved her father and knew that telling her mother would mean the end of her relationship with him. Eventually Cora managed the situation by always taking a friend with her on these weekend visits. (Obviously, this posed a potential danger for the friends. Fortunately, her father restrained himself, rather than approaching Cora's friends.)

When viewed from a distance, without the real-life encumbrances of distraught or contrite parents, the threat of criminal charges, irate attorneys, and a confused child, it should be very obvious that Cora's problem had nothing whatsoever to do with "reporting" her father or "disclosing" his sexual abuse of her. Her problem was her father's behavior and the danger it created for Cora. However, when Cora entered treatment, this clearly was not what she thought. Her idea was that she shouldn't have let the molestation happen in the first place, that she should have stopped it after it started, and that she should have told her mother or someone else. Forgetting that she also abhorred the experience, she blamed herself for enjoying the sexual pleasure so much that she would hide the molestation. After all, she had learned about "bad touch" and was "old enough to know better."

Abused children frequently have good reason to believe that if they talk about being hit, or burned, or participating in sexual activities, their words will *not* be carefully considered. Even if he has not been overtly threatened, the child who lives in a state of chronic but unpredictable violence has an exquisite understanding of the dangers that might arise from his revelations (Herman, 1992). The culture in which children live will also influence their readiness to talk to adults outside the family. For example, children who themselves have been removed or known other children who have been removed from their parents' custody by a social service system or concerned members of an extended family may not only fear retribution and additional harm from their abusers, but they may also hide the abuse from teachers or social workers out of a fear of being separated from their parents. In communities that hold to a "spare the rod and spoil the child" philosophy of child raising, a child whose physical punishment goes beyond the bounds of community norms may be reluctant to talk to adults in positions of authority out of a fear of additional punishment. Or a child in that situation simply may not know that being beaten with an extension cord, locked in a shower of scalding hot water, or having one's head held in a toilet exceeds the bounds of acceptable discipline, even if corporal punishment is the norm within his community.

When children do talk about physical or sexual abuse, it is often not until significantly after the events have taken place. In addition, they typically later retract their stories (Myers, 1992), often supporting their denial with alternative narratives. Thus, the people working with an abused child may be faced with a panoply of stories and memories. Without some understanding of the developmental aspects of memory as well as external factors that affect what and how children remember, those trying to help a child may inadvertently do harm or render themselves ineffectual. For example, if a therapist asks a child leading or coercive questions about suspected abuse, that therapist may render her- or himself useless in any attempts to prosecute the alleged perpetrator (Myers, 1992). Even worse, demanding or suggestive questioning may replicate the coercive experiences that brought the child to treatment.

Ordinarily therapists have the luxury of treating children's memories as they would any other verbal or nonverbal communication. The meaning of both the memory and its introduction into the treatment can be explored at a pace and rhythm determined by child and therapist. So, for example, when 4-year-old Maria announces that she remembers "when she was inside her mommy who was smoking those cigarettes that made her cough and get born and go to the place where you get mommies who know how to take care of kids," I am free to presume that Maria is using this "memory" in trying to make sense of the process that led to her adoption. I am bound by no external requirement to inform anyone of this memory. If Maria had made this same statement to a teacher or parent, they too would have little reason to be concerned about the "truth" of her memory.

However, when a child says that he has been abused, the entire relationship of concerned adults to the child's memory shifts. Suddenly, the accuracy of the child's statement about remembered events can become of greater concern than the meaning of the communication. In work with abused children, it certainly may be necessary or to the child's great advantage if he can recreate, as closely as possible, the events that others consider abusive. For example, in order to be removed from the care of a physically abusive parent, the child may be well served if he can accurately remember and articulate to the investigator where his father keeps the belt used for beatings. The successful prosecution of a pedophile may depend on the ability of his victims to give detailed recounting of the sexual molestation they endured.

However, as we have seen in the false memory debate, in instances when the literal truth is of paramount importance, for example, the prosecution of someone accused of abuse, the parties involved can easily be polarized into two warring camps. There are those who urge great caution in accepting the veracity of children's statements because of research demonstrating the unreliability of children's memories and experiments repeatedly showing that children, as well as adults, can be manipulated into believing in the accuracy of their memory for events that never happened. These arguments are countered by demonstrations of the accuracy of children's memories and experimental evidence that suggests that children resist incorporating false information into their memories (Ceci, Huffman, Smith, & Loftus, 1994; Ceci, Loftus, Leichtman, & Bruck, 1994; Garry & Loftus, 1994; Howe, Courage, & Peterson, 1996; Terr, 1996; Tobey & Goodman, 1992; Spence 1994; Perry, 1995; Pezdek & Roe, 1996; Laub & Auerhahn, 1993; Katz, Schonfeld, Carter, Leventhal, & Cicchetti, 1995; Kihlstrom, 1994; Gordon, Schroeder, Ornstein, & Baker-Ward, 1995). These issues are of particular concern at the time a child initially talks about sexual or physical abuse because that is typically when decisions must be made about whether to remove a child from a presumably abusive situation or to move toward arrest and eventual prosecution of an alleged perpetrator.

There is a great and murky gray area between the position that "children don't lie" about abuse and the position that children can be coached, whether deliberately or inadvertently, into "confessing" all manner of unseemly activities. The interviewer's bias in relation to this continuum will influence the approach he takes in obtaining any additional information from the child or attempting to verify what the child has previously said. For example, some researchers make convincing arguments that moderately leading or suggestive questions are appropriate and sometimes necessary to aid young children in the retrieval of memories. Others would argue that even mildly leading questions run the risk of influencing a child to "remember" what she believes the interviewer wants to hear (Goodman, Quas, Batterman-

Faunce, & Riddlesberger, 1994; Steward, Bussey, Goodman, & Saywitz, 1993; Strichartz & Burton, 1990; Sivan, 1991; Ruffman, Olson, Ash, & Keenan, 1993; Rogers, 1995; Loftus, 1993).

Aparallel debate concerning the believability of children's memories for abuse stems from theories about the ways in which traumatic memories are encoded and retrieved. If, as many argue (Perry, Pollard, Blakley, & Baker, 1995), memory is state-dependent, then the affective experience of terror will result in the attendant sensory images being stored in the subcortical areas of the brain as a series of "flashbulb" images. Unlike memories that undergo modification and structuralization as they are processed by the cerebral cortex, these "autobiographical memories" are characterized by a "frozen" quality, as if the sights, sounds, and smells of the original experiences have been seared into the brain exactly as received. These terror-driven memories are viewed as less vulnerable to the distortions that can and do accompany the encoding of narrative memory. From this understanding of neurobiological processes arises the hypothesis that flashbacks, which are so frequently associated with the traumatic consequences of abuse, are accurate sensory representations of externally generated experiences (Nash, 1994; Ornstein & Myers, 1996) and therefore should be accorded a privileged veridical status. If flashbacks are understood in this way, their presence means that what is stored in memory as a flashback actually happened and is represented to consciousness in an undisturbed form.

Alternatively, if flashbacks are viewed as one of many kinds of memories, all equally subject to modification and distortion, then they hold no special place as representations of reality. From this vantage point, flashbacks are equally likely to depict internally as well as remembering externally generated images. Thus, a child who is immobilized in terror by the sudden intrusive sensation of being strangled may be remembering a dream, a daydream, or a hallucination, as well as the feeling of being suffocated by her mother's hands squeezing her throat. This perspective demands that a flashback be subjected to the same scrutiny as any other memory in order to understand fully the meanings it embodies. A complete exploration would include not only an analysis of the content of the memory, but the timing of its appearance and the importance of any stimulus that seemed to have triggered the particular flashback.

Atherapist's theoretical stance toward the veracity or malleability of memory has profound effects on her attitude toward remembered material that patients bring to therapy. Because of the frequency with which flashbacks have been associated with trauma and posttraumatic stress syndromes (Frankel, 1993; Kluft, 1996; van der Kolk & van der Hart, 1991; van der Kolk, Greenberg, Boyd, & Krystal, 1985), their appearance in clinical material can raise questions that the ordinary memories of childhood do not. If the content of flashbacks has to do with abuse, the therapist who views them as externally generated and primitively encoded memories is likely to accept them as convincing evidence of abuse. The therapist who assumes that flashbacks, like any form of memory, are subject to distortion, may be more concerned with the meaning of the form in which the memory was both stored and retrieved.

Carol

Since midchildhood Carol had struggled with feelings of inadequacy, worthlessness, and depression. Her relationship with her parents was so emotionally bereft that in early adolescence, at the recommendation of her counselor, Carol was sent to live with an older, married sister. Here she felt loved and well cared for, though when she got pulled into the arguments between her sister and brother-in-law she became quite uncomfortable. Carol and her counselor recognized the sexualized nature of her relationship with her brother-in-law, who would often confide in Carol his sexual frustrations with his wife.

In her late 20s Carol again sought psychotherapy because of concerns about her difficulties in sustaining a sexual relationship with her fiancé. From the time she first became sexually active, sexual intercourse made Carol physically and emotionally uncomfortable. She described her fiancé as concerned, caring, and patient and felt that their relationship was good, except that she was so discomfited at the mere thought of intercourse, that she could tolerate virtually no erotic contact. Based on Carol's description of her history and current symptoms, the therapist she consulted suggested that Carol might be suffering the effects of childhood sexual abuse. Though Carol had no conscious memory of sexual abuse prior to this therapy, she had also wondered about that possibility. She and her physician had been unable to find any physical problem that would account for the intense pain and burning she felt on penetration. She also had no ready explanation for the real aversion she felt toward intercourse.

About 1 year into therapy, Carol learned that her brother-in-law was gravely ill. She quickly arranged a trip to visit with him and her sister. Carol was deeply saddened by his condition, felt vaguely uncomfortable during the visit, but returned home with a renewed conviction about his unconditional love for her.

On the first morning following her visit, as she was awakening from a fretful sleep, an unpleasant image of her brother-in-law's face floated above her. She felt her fiancé's hand caressing her breast; at that moment Carol had an intensely unpleasant sensation of a long-forgotten smell of cologne. She bolted from the bed in horror.

By the time she reported this most frightening incident to her therapist, Carol had associated this smell with her brother-in-law. Upon hearing this story, Carol's therapist, with sadness and sympathy, explained how it confirmed their suspicions that Carol's brother-in-law had sexually molested her. Her therapist explained that Carol's terrified response to the intrusive images suggested that she had repressed any memories of her molestation.

Over the next several months, Carol struggled with this revelation, her doubts about the truth it contained, and her worry that her doubts were merely attempts to turn away from the truth. Eventually Carol decided to stop therapy because she "just wasn't getting anywhere." Her therapist felt that Carol's decision to terminate therapy was a resistance to accepting the sad and terrifying reality that the person she had loved most in the world had violated her trust and her body.

During the next year, the brother-in-law's health continued to fail. He asked Carol to come for a visit. She refused, feeling that she just could not be near a man who had molested her. Yet she longed to see him and continued to wonder if he really had molested her. Carol again entered therapy to try to resolve these questions.

The second therapist was less persuaded by the truth contained in the memories Carol described. Over several months of working together, the therapist and Carol began to wonder about what factors might have brought the frightening image of her brother-in-law's face, the smell of cologne, and the terror of her fiancé's sexual touch together.

They considered the impact that several days of sleep deprivation might have had on Carol's state of consciousness. The experience occurred right after a visit to her brother-in-law when the image of his face, along with memories of the sights, sounds, and smells from her childhood, were very present in her mind. She had been in an altered state of consciousness, moving from sleep to wakefulness, when she had experienced this flashback. Her new therapist wondered whether her fiancé's sexual touch had inadvertently stirred some of Carol's old sexual longings for her brother-in-law. Her revulsion might then have been in response to her own feelings rather than in response to a memory of sexual molestation.

Although this analysis also brought into play some anxiety and discomfort, it "felt right" to Carol. For another few months she continued to work with these new ideas and the feelings they stirred. She also addressed her ambivalence about resuming a relationship with her dying brother-in-law, and the inevitably unanswered questions that any important relationship stirs. Ultimately, Carol decided to end therapy, feeling that she had reached her goal of understanding the meaning of a particular memory. Although both she and her therapist felt confident of the analysis they had reached, they acknowledged a slight, but lingering uncertainty about whether they had opted for the more palatable story in order to avoid a horrific truth.

As an adult, Carol had the option of both voicing and acting on her discomfort with her first therapist's diagnosis of childhood sexual abuse. Children typically have few choices; generally, they don't select their own therapists, and if they disagree with a diagnosis, they may be less free to voice that opinion, particularly if doing so is taken as evidence that they have not yet accepted the reality of abuse, or if they are caught between warring parents.

Since we know that children can and will defend even the most abusive parent almost to the death, therapists are regularly called upon to make judgments about whether a child is protecting an abusive parent, disclosing the realities of living with physical or sexual abuse, or making statements that have more to do with internal than external realities. It certainly happens that, at the same time that children are verbally denying having been abused, their play may tell a quite different story. Yet, play themes, like all else in psychotherapy, are open to interpretation, and therapists, like everyone else, are vulnerable to seeing what they are looking for in both the process and content of play.

Therefore, especially when there is a possibility of abuse in the child's life, those who treat children absolutely must exercise vigilance about the biases we bring to our work. We must rigorously and continually monitor our formulations and emotional responses in order to ensure, as best we can, that we are responding to the material the child brings to therapy rather than letting other factors impinge on our therapeutic work. This admirable goal is easy to embrace in theory, but when an anxious mother is begging her child's therapist to make the court stop visits to the father, an irate father is demanding support for his position that the child be moved into his home in order to avoid being brainwashed by the mother, and the court wants advice about how to handle the situation, even the most well-intentioned and seasoned clinician may have difficulty protecting the therapeutic space against the external pressures to find clarity prematurely or certainty where none exists. Psychotherapy demands that we, with the child, tolerate *not knowing*. Only from this position, in which all of the child's material is accepted for exploration and understanding, can true analytic exploration and understanding take place.

Maya

Maya's parents' divorce, when she was about 7, involved extensive, ugly accusations between her parents. Her mother accused her father of sexual perversion; the father alleged that the mother was a man-hating lesbian. Each accused the other of drug and alcohol abuse. Both admitted to prior substance abuse, but each claimed to be "clean and sober" at the time they were trying to settle custody and visitation issues. The parents agreed to the mother's having primary physical custody of Maya with the child spending every other weekend with her father.

This plan worked reasonably well for a few months until Maya returned home from a weekend visit with her father saying she didn't want to go back because she "didn't like what he did." Other than adding that she "just felt weird and stuff," Maya would say no more. She became increasingly agitated when her mother probed for more information.

When her mother confronted her father with Maya's complaints, she thought he sounded drunk or stoned during the conversation. He denied that there was any reason for Maya to stop weekend visits, complaining that his ex-wife was "a man-hating bitch" who thought even a father's giving his daughter a good-night kiss was perverted.

Alarmed, the mother filed a report with Children's Protective

Services and contacted her attorney. The court ordered a custody evaluation and required Maya's visits with her father to be supervised in the interim. Rather than allaying the mother's fears, this recommendation intensified her concerns. She worried that the supervisor, a friend and former drinking buddy of the father's would, at best, cover up the molestation of her daughter and, at worst, participate in it.

During this period, Maya became increasingly unwilling to talk to her mother about visits with her father. Fearing that Maya had been coerced into hiding something, her mother initiated family therapy for herself, her new partner, and Maya. In the course of the evaluation, the therapist suggested that Maya bring the clothes that she had been wearing at the time of the suspected molestation. The therapist explained that wearing the same clothes sometimes helped children to remember exactly what had occurred and to recreate the feelings they had had during any traumatic event.

The therapist further suggested that Maya be dressed for her therapy sessions in the clothes that she had worn during each most recent visit with her father. The mother had come to feel quite certain that the father had fondled Maya during the routine of putting her to bed. She based her opinion on Maya's recent insistence on wearing only pajamas to bed, the father's comment about the good-night kiss, and Maya's affirmative nod when she was asked if her father had ever touched her "there" (genital area). This question was asked while her mother was drying Maya's genital area after a bath.

Sometimes Maya protested wearing the assigned clothes; sometimes she said that Daddy didn't touch her; sometimes she said she "didn't want to talk about it." The therapist felt that this confusion was consistent with the behavior of children who have been sexually abused. Following each visit with her father, Maya was asked to show her mother and the therapist all of the places that Daddy had touched her clothing. She never touched her genital area.

Meanwhile, the evaluator completed the custody evaluation. The evaluator concluded that Maya's father had indeed resumed a pattern of excessive drinking, which the father reluctantly admitted to. The evaluator felt that Maya was so anxious about her father's drinking even "a beer at a Christmas party" that her worry about that might account for her "feeling weird and stuff." He recommended that the father enter an alcohol treatment program and begin therapy to address some broad issues of impulse control. He concluded that it was impossible for Maya to think or speak clearly about the reason(s) for her discomfort in her father's presence because both her mother and therapist were convinced that Maya *had* been molested by her father. Although the evaluator felt that Maya's mother's concerns were exaggerated, in the interests of protecting both Maya and her father, he recommended that the father's friend, who was considered a reputable member of the community, continue to monitor the visits for 6 months. He suggested a reassessment at that time.

After several months, Maya and her mother moved to a neighboring community, which made the commute to therapy quite difficult. Although they tried to continue, eventually there were just too many missed sessions, and the mother and therapist agreed that Maya should have therapy in her new community.

The new relationship got off to a rocky start when the therapist insisted on meeting with the father as well as the mother. Maya's mother expressed her concern that the father was such a "smooth talker" that the therapist would believe his lies that he had never touched his daughter inappropriately. She was extremely suspicious of the whole idea since the previous therapist had never met with the father because that "would make Maya feel that therapy was not a safe place."

Prior to Maya's first visit to the new therapist, her mother had called to report exactly what Maya had said when she returned from the visit and to explain that they would be a little late because she had to get Maya home to change into her weekend clothes, even though the new therapist had said that, as far as he was concerned, Maya could wear whatever she wanted to the appointment. After the session, the mother called to find out exactly what he had asked and what Maya had said about being molested. The therapist repeated his request to have a few sessions to get to know Maya before speaking with Maya's parents about his recommendations. He reminded the mother that if he had any reason to believe that Maya was in danger he would do whatever was necessary to ensure her safety.

In the first session with Maya, the therapist had told her that he knew that people were worried about whether her father had touched her in ways that made her uncomfortable; he said that this was something they could think about together if she wanted. Maya responded by proceeding with her activity as if he had not spoken. The therapist found Maya a relatively contained little girl who played readily but spoke little.

At the end of the evaluation period, the therapist concluded that he really could not definitely state whether Maya had been molested. He reassured her mother that there was nothing in Maya's conversation or play that made him concerned that she was currently in danger; that he felt he could be helpful to Maya by allowing her to bring up the things she felt were important; and that it would likely take quite a while for Maya to get to know and trust him.

The mother expressed her dismay at this news. The therapist had merely confirmed Maya's report that he "only wanted to play." At that point, Maya's mother concluded that the new therapist was inept and that she would have to resign herself to driving the considerable distance to Maya's previous therapist.

This story contains a number of disturbing elements, the most important being the possibility that this child had been subjected to sexual abuse by her father and/or his friend but could not let anyone know for certain about it. While the mother's anxiety clearly included some pathological elements, it also stemmed, at least in part, from her concern for her child's well-being and her sense that her daughter returned distressed after visits with her father. The psychologist who conducted the evaluation had sufficient concern about the child's safety to recommend supervision, but he entertained enough doubt about the allegations that he did not recommend against visits. The first therapist's interest in "helping the child remember" abusive events grew out of a conviction that empowering a child to stop the abuse was the primary goal of therapy. And, like the evaluating psychologist, the second therapist was uncertain about what, if any, harm had come to this child during one or more visits to her father.

One unfortunate outcome of the focus on getting this child to remember and reveal what really happened was that it quite likely contributed to her silence, thereby making it impossible to determine if she had been or currently was in danger. She was silent not only about what occurred during her visits with her father, but about her emotional life before, during, and after those visits. Because the mother and the first therapist were so focused on what the father might have done to Maya, they missed the opportunity to hear Maya's subjective experiences of her father—the interactions, longings, disappointments, memories, and distortions. When this therapist set the stage for Maya to remember and demonstrate the abuse, she made it clear, whether implicitly or explicitly, that she was interested only in some of Maya's memories, only in certain aspects of Maya, thus conveying to Maya that she was, first and foremost, an abused child, whether or not she admitted it. The goal of the therapy was for Maya to retrieve a memory about the actions of another, so that she could employ "the truth" to change the facts of her life. Perhaps Maya understood that both her mother and her therapist wanted to hear only their idea of the correct version of the truth, or perhaps Maya was silent because she had a different version of the truth. However, Maya really might have been molested by her father, but because her mother was not affectively attuned to her subjective experience, Maya quite literally had nothing to say. Her mother's clarity and certainty about what surely happened perhaps heightened Maya's sense of confusion and ambiguity of memory. Perhaps Maya interpreted the request for a clear statement as an indication that nothing else was worth speaking.

Indeed, the second therapist who saw Maya found that almost any topic was one she "didn't want to talk about," although she eagerly played with the dollhouse. Much of her play concerned confused and affectively charged separations and reunions. The interactions among the dolls were repetitiously brutal but not sexualized. Unfortunately, before he had time to learn what, if anything, about physical, sexual, or emotional abuse might be embedded in Maya's play, their relationship ended.

The therapist who is primarily interested in the child's psychological truth is aware that while the events that brought the abused child to treatment cannot be changed, no matter how much both child and therapist may wish it, the child's understanding of those events can and will be altered over time. Does this mean that a child who says one day that Daddy hit her and the next that he didn't is one day lying and the next telling the truth, or one day telling the truth and the next day "covering" for a parent, or too frightened to tell what *really* happened? Of course we want to know; however, of greater importance for the therapy is the recognition that the child has a complex story to tell and that her understanding of the events in her life is variable.

Memories are more or less accessible for a wide range of reasons, not all of which involve coercion or anxiety. For example, we have all had the experience of a distinct memory being triggered by an external stimulus. Even though the memory might have been accessible in the moment before it arose, it was not in consciousness.

While children can sometimes give clear and straightforward accounts of their experiences, abuse often takes place under circumstances that contribute to a child's confusion about what is really happening, let alone why. Physical abuse may occur in the midst of a raging parent's tirade against the child, the other parent, or other children in the family. The child may have a clear memory of what caused the outburst or may remember a "reason" in order to make sense of an otherwise senseless scene. Certainly children sometimes "invent" reasons for brutal punishment, rather than accept their helplessness in the face of an unpredictably violent parent. In the case of sexual molestation, the abusive events may take place when the child is already in an altered state of consciousness. As the following cases illustrate, the consequent uncertainties and confusion may contribute to the child's difficulties talking to those who might stop the molestation or otherwise help her.

Cora

Cora was often "half asleep" when her father would slip into her bed at night and fondle her genitals. Part of Cora's reluctance to talk about this stemmed from her initial confusion about whether this was a dream or a memory. Since she wasn't sure, she was afraid of being told that she was making it up or that she had "dirty" thoughts. Because her father's attentions also gave her pleasure, Cora felt guilty both about her pleasure and about not telling anyone. The longer she put off asking for help, the guiltier she felt; the intensity of her guilt eventually left her unable to turn to anyone for help.

If a child has consciously or unconsciously relied heavily on dissociation to manage the horror of abuse, she may have great difficulty in telling someone what "really" happened.

Jackie

Jackie, a young girl of 18, described feeling nauseated by certain chewing or "smacking" sounds. She had no idea what was so disturbing about these noises, but she found them so intolerable that she would have to leave the room if she happened to be in the presence of a particularly noisy eater. Jackie had vague memories of having been sexually molested as a very young child by an upstairs neighbor, but her recollections of the sexual activities themselves were fuzzy. One evening, the sounds made by a man seated behind her in a movie theater left her flooded with a queasy recognition that the sound was of her abuser's performing oral sex on her. She then had a memory of wondering why he would want to "eat" her, a thought that made her sick. Jackie recalled no genital or vaginal sensations either during the abuse itself or in response to the chewing sounds that had tormented her.

Jackie did not remember telling her parents about these events, feeling that she really didn't know what to say. Even though the specifics of the molestation were not available to conscious memory, Jackie knew that she really didn't like this neighbor and didn't want to be around him, but rather than tell her parents why or ask for their help, she found ways to avoid him.

Betty

Betty, who began psychotherapy in late adolescence, tried to explain why she had never told her parents about the abuse she had suffered at the hands of a family friend:

> "What do you say to your mother? I was little. I didn't know at first what it was. I didn't have any words. And then you go to school and you learn the words from the kids. I thought, 'That's it. That's what he's doing.' But when you learn the words you know you don't say them to your mother. 'Fuck?' I was supposed to say that to my mother?!"

She didn't. Instead, for years she tried both consciously and unconsciously by her behavior to tell her parents that something terrible had happened to her, something unspeakable and that, as a result, something was dreadfully wrong. They didn't listen. They, like Paul's parents, behaved as if there were nothing amiss, as if there were no Korean War on the top of the barn.

As a result, for a while, Betty put her ideas aside, thinking maybe the feelings, intrusive memories, and terrifying dreams would just somehow disappear. Later, she believed that her parents actually, though unconsciously, knew what they didn't want to hear or see. She felt that the evidence was too powerful, that they were too smart, too savvy about such things. Yet Betty sensed that verbalizing, putting words to her story, would be too disruptive. She anticipated that her parents would be wounded, that they wouldn't know what to say. She feared that their lives would come apart because all of their friendships would be affected. In essence, it would just be a big mess.

Betty was not a fool. She knew that her fears about the effects of disclosure on these interpersonal relationships were based in reality, but she also came to recognize a defensive aspect to her rhetoric. *She herself* didn't want to know about the abuse. She loathed naming it, because to do so would be to give it meaning.

Paradoxically, it would also destroy the unreality in which she had tried to live for so many years. Without language to describe and order these memories, they did not seem entirely real to Betty. Although she did not refer to the underlying neurological processes, Betty's descriptions of these fragmented images vividly describe the subjective experience of "remembering" events that have not been subjected to cortical processing. These memories, apparently stored in the more primitive areas of the brain, remained frozen in her mind in the time and space in which they occurred. They had not been organized or integrated, either cognitively or affectively, by thought, language, or meaningful associations, into higher levels of cortical memory (see Chapter 4). Betty resisted doing this because she recognized that really "thinking" about the abuse would result in truly knowing what had happened to her. However, she also came to understand that only by allowing herself to think—that is, to bring cortical organization to these images—could she control them and regulate the attendant affects.

At this point in her life, Betty's self-image was structured around her view of herself as an abused child. She attempted to rid herself of that internalized self-representation in a quite simple and completely ineffectual manner: "If I just don't say it, it won't be true." So, even though she consciously and fervently wished that her parents would learn of her molestation and punish the perpetrator, Betty was deeply ambivalent about her parents' failure to recognize or name the source of her misery. She simultaneously wanted them to know without having to tell them and felt relief when they didn't seem to recognize what was wrong. If they, also, didn't say it, perhaps "it" truly wasn't real. Alternatively, perhaps she could still hope they would recognize a truth she found too painful to verbalize.

Betty's parents did know that she was an unhappy child. She recalled their numerous failed attempts to understand and mitigate her depression and general sense of unease. They tried summer camp, a

change of schools, various classes and lessons. They even tried psychotherapy. Despite these interventions, Betty did not get any happier and
did not verbalize what she wanted her parents to know. Increasingly,
she appeared to herself, her teachers, and parents a sullen and willfully
unhappy child. She claimed they didn't understand her; they agreed
and asked why she wouldn't tell them what was wrong. Throughout
her childhood, Betty's parents maintained a continuous, though not
close, relationship with the man who molested her. Betty experienced
this as both a betrayal and as a periodic source of temporary relief,
wishing that her parents' acceptance of this acquaintance meant that
he could not be a person who would hurt their child or that, through
their contact with him, his true character and aberrant behavior would
reveal themselves.

Unfortunately, each time Betty's parents responded to her seemingly incomprehensible behavior or statements that they did not
understand her they confirmed her internalized image of them as
extremely adept with words but terrified of feelings. When they looked
to experts or outside activities for help in alleviating her depression,
Betty interpreted their behavior as evidence that they could not
tolerate knowing the facts or feelings of her molestation.

Like many abused children, Betty found herself in a psychologically untenable position. Though her parents were capable people,
prominent in their fields, and determined in their efforts to be good
parents, Betty's internalized representations were of ineffectual parents. She saw her father's facility with words as providing him an
easy avenue for distancing himself from emotional difficulties; she
felt her mother's psychological stability as resting on a carefully
controlled, superficial tranquillity in all of their relationships. Betty
feared that the underlying emotional fragility could not bear the
weight of powerful affect. In relation to these internalized objects,
Betty felt herself to be "too much"—too damaged, too scared, and
too sad to be truly known by them. She could not turn inward,
relying on the internalized parental representations for comfort, nor
did her internalized world of object relations allow her to look to
her actual parents for help.

Essentially, Betty spent her childhood waiting for her parents to
transform themselves into the parents she wanted them to be—parents
who were empathically attuned to her, who could recognize and
tolerate her pain without being overwhelmed or turning away. Her
dilemma lay in her idea that only in *not* telling them could she

preserve the hope that they would actually behave in ways that she wanted and needed, yet in keeping silent, she perpetuated her image of them as inept parents who could not possibly help her. Betty did not tell her parents about being molested because, in her mind, doing so would only result in disappointment and further despair, destroying the potential for actualizing the wished-for parents of her internal world. Of equal importance was her conviction that they would feel despair and inadequacy in response to her disclosures; they were not bad people or unfeeling parents. She could not bear to see them wracked with guilt over having failed to protect her. The thought of their crumbling in the face of her disclosure was more than she could bear.

When we counterpoise Betty's memories of years-long struggle over how and what to tell her parents against Alice's memory of a relatively easy request for parental help in a similarly difficult situation, the contrast will strike us painfully. Certainly in considering the distinctions, we must take into account the age difference—Alice was in early adolescence when she was approached by the family employee, while Betty was probably a preschooler. However, age, developmental sophistication, or cognitive capacities do not fully account for Alice's revelation or Betty's silence. Adolescents do suffer unwanted sexual advances in silence and 3- and 4-year-olds can and do say, "I don't like him," or "He hurts me," or "I don't want to go there."

These two stories illuminate the crucial role of internalized images of self and object in the disclosure of childhood abuse. Alice asked for help because she expected to get it. As a result, she was left with a narrative available to conscious memory. Her story had a beginning, middle, and end; its construction allowed her to consciously contain an ambivalently held object in an integrated memory from her childhood.

Unfortunately, Betty did not fare so well. Her object relationships, stemming perhaps in part from developmental immaturity, did not allow her to get the help she needed in stopping the sexual molestation at its inception. As a result, she was left with disorganized and dissociated fragments of intrusive part-memories that her words were inadequate to describe. Her relationship to her parents remained locked in the world of action with all of its imprecision and opportunities for misinterpretations. She remained sullen, unhappy, and beyond their understanding; they remained confused, ineffectual, uncomprehending.

When we approach memories as living constructs, rather than as pristinely preserved artifacts, we recognize both the futility of a search for historical truth and the certainty that any memories of abuse will inevitably become an integral part of the therapeutic work. Abusive experiences are in the child's brain and mind; she can no more eliminate them from her being than she can other aspects of herself. They may show themselves clearly in her play, or she may tell us plainly in words about exactly what happened to her; alternatively, she may go to extraordinary lengths to conceal the abusive experiences from herself and exclude them from the therapeutic relationship. As with abuse itself, the effects may be blatant or subtle.

Although external pressures often lead us to believe that we cannot offer effective psychotherapy unless we know for sure the details of a child's past, we must protect the child's right to uncertainty and privilege her moving toward insight at a pace she sets for herself. For our purposes *whether* children remember abusive experiences in a historically accurate way is less important than *how* they show and tell us about themselves. Even when children struggle against integrating abusive experiences, the effects of these events will become evident if we pay careful attention to the feelings, words, and actions children use to either reveal or hide them. Research on neurological and psychological aspects of memory, the consequences of trauma, and normative development processes offer us powerful tools for recognizing the consequences of abuse in the behavior and affective interchanges of the children who come to us for treatment. Simultaneously, we must accept that we cannot always know for certain whether a child has been abused and that we will demean both the therapeutic process and the child's experience of uncertainty if we attempt to influence him, whether overtly or covertly, into disclosing or denying that he has been a victim of child abuse.

Chapter Six

Looking Outward: Externalization and Dissociation

Children often make prodigious efforts to keep both the facts and power of abuse as something separate from themselves. Adults, who understandably wish the abuse, whether suffered at the hands of family, friend, or stranger, not to have a lasting impact on their child, frequently support their efforts. Unfortunately, what caretakers and children often want, but don't always state openly, is that the child be restored to a pristine "preabuse" condition—the abuse to be undone, never to have happened.

Paradoxically, these strategies only intensify the psychological power of abusive experiences. The patient suffering from paranoia is inevitably pursued by external enemies because his unacceptable impulses and feelings are projected onto, or assigned, to others. Thus he feels that others, over whom he has no control, threaten him; he does not understand that mastery of the danger he feels will come only after he accepts the impulses and feelings as his own. The same holds for the child who has tried to escape the effects of abuse by resisting internalization. Instead of mastering the trauma, she condemns herself to a lasting sense of herself, both in her mind and the minds of those close to her, as someone damaged by forces beyond her control—an irreparable victim of child abuse.

The relationship between dissociative defenses and overwhelming psychic trauma has been well established from both research and clinical perspectives (Bremner, Krystal, Charney, & Southwick, 1996; Bromberg, 1996; Davies & Frawley, 1991; Gleaves, 1996; Hartman & Burgess, 1993; Krystal, 1990; Mulhern, 1994; Putnam, 1988, 1993; Watkins & Watkins, 1990). In the present context, I would like to consider one aspect of dissociation, namely, its effectiveness in helping the victim of abuse maintain an external focus. Whether consciously or unconsciously initiated, a dissociated state has to do with psychological departure from the source of pain.

One young woman described her efforts to remove herself as "going out the window." In anticipation of an impending sexual assault, she would do psychologically what she could not do physically—simply leave. While we easily recognize this as a dissociative process, I want to emphasize that the dissociation serves the attempt to keep the abusive experience from entering psychic reality. The dissociative state may be consciously invoked in order to shield the self from a psychologically unfathomable and unmanageable experience, as if the child is saying, "I can't stop this from happening to my body, but I can stop it from happening to *me*." In this sense, the self becomes disembodied, and the body is then experienced as not only separate from the self, but as external to the self. It becomes, in essence a part of the external world.

Though the definitions and descriptions of dissociation vary, it is clinically useful to consider dissociation as an interplay of psychological and physiological processes resulting in a psychological state(s) in which an event is experienced and stored in memory as a shattered image. When a child responds to a perceived danger by a heightened state of arousal of the subcortical areas of the brain, the higher-order neurological processes, which typically bring complex thought, order, meaning, and affective modulation to experience, are inhibited (see Chapter 4). Events experienced in this manner are retained in the same way, as unintegrated, fragmented sensations that are "dis-associated" from each other and from the child's cohesively experienced sense of herself. Even if some aspects of an experience are remembered, some of its elements, if they are simply too painful to be available to conscious awareness, may be held in a dissociated state. The disorganized pictures that frequently characterize these states resemble an unassembled jigsaw puzzle; all of the pieces are there, but the fragmentation prevents the cohesiveness of remembered experience. The eventual picture that will emerge from the scattered colors and forms of the puzzle may be more or less recognizable, depending on how many, how small, and how scrambled the pieces. If an event is too painful to be endured consciously, if it overwhelms the capacity of the ego to comprehend and integrate it, then dissociation, or a psychological movement into a parallel state of consciousness, may be the mind's final attempt to avoid disintegration into psychosis.

Esther, who began psychotherapy in adolescence, described routinely waking from dreams in sweaty terror. The nightmares that tormented her contained no monsters, no personifications of evil pursuers; rather they were flashes, blinding, racing fragments of feelings. She knew these dreams concerned the sexual abuse she had suffered as a child. Though they were horrifying, she was even more fearful of allowing the pieces to become integrated into a cohesive picture. She recognized that any such picture would be inside her; if she put the pieces together, the image would be of her making. Just as a photograph is not a simple duplication of a scene, but the creation of the photographer, the fragmented, dissociated pieces that are used to maintain abuse as external become internalized as they become coherent.

Like many defensive strategies, dissociation occurs normatively in early development; indeed, parents often encourage it to help children get through difficult moments. For example, when a child is about to get a frightening injection, his sympathetic parent may suggest, "Just think about the ice cream cone we're going to get on the way home." If the child can successfully remove himself from the painful stimulus, that is, if he has disassociated himself from a frightening situation, then his memory of the experience will be quite different from that of the child who remained cognitively and affectively present during the experience. His memory for the event may be vague or confused; though he may be able to articulate that he "got a shot," when pressed about his internal experience, he may well find it difficult to say exactly what happened, precisely because he wasn't entirely there! He knows what happened *to* him, but not what happened *in* him. Dissociation serves quite effectively to resist the internalization and integration of unpleasant experiences. However, when one has not been wholly present during an experience, when one part of the self has been removed in order to manage the terror or pain, there is no cohesive whole available to conscious memory. There is no continuous, coherent story to hold in the self or to convey to another.

While we can relatively easily define and distinguish among defenses for semantic purposes, in the real world of evaluation and treatment, defenses show themselves in clusters and cannot always be so easily separated, particularly when they are working simultaneously, one enhancing or enabling another. For example, at first glance, it might seem that dissociation and obsessive–compulsive behavior are quite different defensive strategies that could be easily distinguished. But consider the child who carefully lines up a bin of cars and trucks and repetitively and compulsively counts each and every one. During this activity, he appears to go into a trance-like state and seems to be utterly unaware of his surroundings. Does the counting induce a dissociative state? If so, is it deliberately used for that purpose, or is it largely a consequence of a sometimes pathologically intense focus? Or might the counting be triggered by a shift into a dissociative state in which the capacity for narrative structure is lost, leaving the child with little other than rote, repetitive activity to ward off intrusive, chaotic images? Any of these is theoretically possible.

In the treatment of a child who has been abused, the pull to focus on the external world poses a particularly sensitive and difficult issue (Novick & Novick, 1994). The abused child has a powerful defensive wish to maintain the event(s) as external, as something that happened *to* him rather than *within* him and thus, to look for external solutions. So, the little boy who arranges and counts his trucks behaves *as if* the disorganization that plagues him is in the external world. He doesn't recognize that putting words to the feelings will begin to bring order both to the neurological pathways that control the modulation of his feelings and to his subjective experience of his inner life (see Chapter 7).

Frequently the child's wish is abetted by the adults around him, who understandably hope that the whole ugly mess can somehow just be made to disappear with no lasting effects. Sometimes their externalization shows itself relatively straightforwardly, as it did with Ruby's aunt (see Chapter 7) who often focused more attention on Ruby's bald spots than on the anxieties that drove her literally to rub the hair right off of her head. In other cases, externalization and displacement combine to create a maddeningly irrelevant sense of moral outrage. A mother who "hadn't noticed" that her boyfriend routinely had sex with her preschool daughter until she saw blood flooding from the child's vagina, developed an almost obsessive concern about having only organic fruit served at the therapeutic nursery school the child later attended. Whether in relatively benign or more insidious ways, these attitudes support the child's beliefs that her troubles lie outside, rather than within.

The impact of abuse cannot be treated successfully until the abuse is understood and accepted by the victim as an internal experience, that is, an event originating externally, intruding itself upon preexisting fantasy, cognitive capabilities, and object relationships. Thus, a thorough investigation of the motivations for and mechanisms that support this external focus is crucial. Just as medical treatment cannot erase the fact of a physical trauma, psychotherapy cannot eradicate the fact of a psychological trauma, but both interventions can and do aim to minimize the trauma's potentially crippling and lasting effects.

Ironically, the child's very efforts to save himself from the consequences of abuse put him in the greatest psychological danger. All of the mechanisms that support this outward focus, and there are many, have as a single aim ensuring the integrity of the nonabused self. Unfortunately, the more tenaciously the child clings to these defensive strategies, the more likely his identity will become structured around the abuse. The mere fact of trying to keep it out of psychic life results in its usurping a primary role in identity formation. Derisha provides a heartbreaking example of the pernicious effects of this process.

Derisha

Almost everyone who knew her saw Derisha as a bright, funny, energetic young woman with a fierce dedication to improving the lot of those less fortunate than she. She worked hard at anything she undertook, was a loyal friend, and seemed to enjoy the many pleasures that life presented her. She felt that her considerable intelligence and sardonic sense of humor contributed to her ease in "fooling" people. She made them think that she was "just like everyone else." When they seemed to accept this lie, she hated them. When people saw through the facade, she dropped them—unless she had determined that they, too, had been victims of child abuse.

Derisha entered therapy when she felt that she was about to lose her mind. In the first session she announced that, although she was relatively certain that she had been subjected to sexual assaults by a family friend from about the ages of 6 to 8, she did not want this to be a primary topic of discussion. She wanted the therapist to understand that she had worked very hard at overcoming these events in order to ensure that they had no impact on her life or on the lives of her immediate family. She hated this man for what he had done to her as a child and had determined that he would not have any effect on her adult life.

The image that Derisha presented to others truly belied her internal world and her view of herself. Throughout high school and college, most of Derisha's relationships—with men and women, with friends and lovers—had involved some element of abuse. A boyfriend beat her; a girlfriend stole money from her and blamed the misbehavior on Derisha, whom she described as "too uptight to lend money to a friend in need." Derisha routinely drank to excess and frequently tried to calm herself with illicit drugs. She suffered from attacks of anxiety, insomnia, nightmares, and suicidal preoccupations. However, her pervasive sense of detachment and disconnection troubled her the most.

Early in life Derisha had determined that she absolutely would *not* become one of the "statistics" of child abuse, that is, that she would not identify herself as a victim. In many external ways, she achieved her goals—she earned the respect of her teachers and colleagues, the admiration of those she supervised, and the devotion and loyalty of friends. Yet, she remained leery of the motives of anyone who approached her as a whole and lovely person.

Ironically and painfully, despite her best conscious efforts to avoid seeing herself as a victim of child abuse, unconsciously she invited continued abuse from the external world. These ongoing hurts confirmed her powerful unconscious identification of herself as a person damaged by abuse. Fortunately, as therapy helped her to integrate the feelings and ideas that stemmed from the abuse, Derisha could begin to protect herself from continued harm.

This vignette shows why a primary task of treatment of abused children is to keep open a full range of possibilities for identification. In doing so, treatment diminishes the likelihood that the person abused as a child will define him- or herself (consciously or not) primarily as a victim of child abuse.

Abused children rely on many, frequently overlapping defenses in their often futile attempts to find comfort and support. These defensive strategies have in common an external focus. The need for the abused child to keep her attention directed toward the outer world has two primary determinants. The first concerns her assessment of real danger emanating from the world around her; the second concerns the absence of a protective internal object to whom she can turn for comfort.

If we are going to help children look inward, we must first appreciate with them the real and imagined dangers they fear will beset them if they turn their attention away from the external world. After all, if one must navigate through a combat zone, it may not be the best time to pause to reflect on the meaning of that experience. When we prematurely ask children to consider feelings and meaning, we lose the opportunity to understand their judgments about the environment and how those impressions inform their behavior. The abused child who is constantly on the alert to external dangers is, in many cases, demonstrating a well-developed sense of reality testing.

In trying to help a child recognize and understand his wish to look outward, rather than inward, the therapist may easily slip into a unidimensional approach. A focus on the child's capacities and needs in the assessment of external dangers and attention to the lack of a stable internal object both draw the child's attention to the external world. Whereas the intricacies of the child's internal life are often more compelling to psychoanalytic clinicians, we simply must not neglect the realities of the child's perceived need to maintain his vigilant stance.

Sam

Seven-year-old Sam learned early that his father's bizarre rages and crying jags were tied to his father's drinking binges. Clearly, it was important for him to pay attention to his father's alcohol intake and to recognize the signs of intoxication in order to maximize the chances of protecting himself from physical harm. Because Sam's father's drinking occurred almost exclusively on paydays, Sam could, with great accuracy predict when his father would arrive home drunk. He learned to avoid his father on those evenings, sometimes by going to his room or, whenever he could, to his grandparents' home. Partly because he was very bright and had unusually well-developed impulse control, Sam also successfully learned to avoid doing or saying things he knew would antagonize his drunken father. It upset him that his older brother did not seem to be as clever as he and frequently ended up in a fight with their father.

Obviously, the eternal vigilance Sam relied on to avoid beatings or verbal humiliation came at a very high psychic price, but because he, unlike his brother, succeeded in protecting himself from his father's attacks, his assessment that he was quite able to fend for himself was to a certain extent realistic. Not surprisingly, he saw little need for therapy; he did not reject or show anger at the therapist's offers, he just didn't really see the point. After all, he didn't feel endangered—and he knew quite well how to avoid problems. He explained to his therapist that "all you had to do was figure out when something bad was going to happen and stay out of the way." He spent many sessions proudly demonstrating his strategies for predicting everything from natural disasters to the outcome of sporting events. Although compulsive and clearly tinged with anxiety, Sam manifested a truly impressive ability to obtain, order, and assess information about the world around him. However, his defensive need to find order and absolute predictability, even where it didn't exist, had robbed him of the chance to appreciate uncertainty and surprise. Sam did not understand that he had expanded his originally useful ability to predict into a world view based on a meaningless consistency. The danger no longer resided solely in the father, who was usually kind and loving but sometimes bizarre, abusive, and embarrassingly remorseful. Sam's need for absolute predictability had now metamorphosed into a constricting attempt to manage the turbulence of affect surrounding the internalized father–child relationship.

Susan

All children look for consistent behavior from their parents, but children of abusive parents often assume predictability in an effort to ease their terror in the face of entirely erratic behavior. Such was the case for Susan, who by the age of 9 had developed a complex ritual that she used to gauge her mother's moods. She explained that, though she often intuited the afternoon's atmosphere the minute she returned home from school, sometimes she had more difficulty discerning her mother's state of mind. If her mother screamed at her when she walked in, things would be bad until her father's arrival home from work brought some relief. If her mother was in bed with a headache, she could probably spend the afternoon alone in her room. Those were the easy days. The hardest days were those when her mother was up and about, perhaps in the kitchen awaiting Susan's arrival. Susan said she could sometimes tell if it would be a bad day by a kind of faraway look in her mother's eyes. If that didn't work, she had a series of questions she would ask and, depending on the answers, decide whether to stay home or try to find an excuse to go to a friend's until dinnertime.

While beautifully crafted, this elaborate plan was not as reliable as Susan liked to believe. Sometimes her mother didn't stay in bed for the afternoon but awoke in a rage. Sometimes the anger that greeted Susan at the door subsided, and mother and daughter could spend a calm afternoon together. At the beginning of therapy Susan explained these anomalies as either lapses in her vigilance—she must have missed a clue—or a flaw in her scheme, meaning that she needed to add a question or change how she asked an existing question. Susan's superficial self-sufficiency in the face of her mother's unpredictable moods and behavior represented a valiant attempt to protect herself from an actual external danger; for when in her worst moods, the mother would hit Susan, as well as scream at her, for any infraction of the "rules"—or, as Susan sadly came to recognize, "for no particular reason at all."

Like Sam, Susan paid a very high price for the protective maneuvers she relied on to shield her from a sense of overwhelming helplessness in the face of her mother's largely erratic mood swings. Unfortunately, because she sometimes could correctly assess her mother's emotional state, she erroneously concluded that absolute accuracy was possible. When Susan began therapy, she couldn't allow herself to know that the problem belonged to her mother. Instead, she blamed herself for her inattentiveness or lack of cleverness and was quite critical of her perceived inability to think clearly. She approached her therapist as a tutor who could help her learn better strategies for gauging her mother's moods. Ambiguity and uncertainty most assuredly did not intrigue this little girl; she wanted answers, not more questions.

Even when a child no longer has contact with the person who hurt him, his hypervigilant stance toward the world often continues.

Although the person who harmed him has been removed from the outer environment, the abuse has become embedded both neurologically and psychologically in the child's experience of himself and his world. If an external danger prompted his fear, anxiety, or inability to concentrate, when those symptoms continued, it would make sense for him to keep his eyes and ears attuned, to remain on the lookout for clues of impending threats. In many instances, the abuse intensifies the child's propensity to project his own aggression into the external world—to fear the monsters in the closet, rather than know the monstrousness of the feelings he carries inside. In other cases, the abuse alerts children to previously unrecognized dangers. If, long after the abuse ends, the child acts as if the danger continues, his behavior may stem from his heightened attention to the external world. What looks like a breakdown in reality testing may actually demonstrate his acute assessment of his real situation.

Max

Max was 6 when his distraught parents sought consultation. They were concerned that Max, who had previously been a calm, easy-going, affectionate child, had become nervous, emotionally labile, and overly concerned about any variation in his routine, misplaced item, or tiny injury. They felt that Max had changed dramatically about 6 months earlier, in response to being sexually molested by a baby-sitter. The sitter had been reported to the police and fired immediately. Max had seemed relieved by his parents' swift response. That Billy was now in jail and couldn't hurt little boys anymore, which was his interpretation of the events that transpired after he talked to the police, pleased Max.

Max had been seen for crisis intervention immediately following the report of abuse. The parents felt that this therapist usefully served both them and Max. They reportedly appreciated her help in understanding Max's symptoms and took seriously her insistence that Max would need their support and reassurance as he struggled to overcome feelings of betrayal, helplessness, and vulnerability.

Immediately following the abuse, Max became extremely demanding of his mother's attention, following her everywhere. His questions about whether his parents were certain that Billy was in jail alternated with pronouncements of his absolute certainty that Billy would stay in jail "forever." Gradually Max's nightmares and questions about Billy subsided, but his persistent questions about his mother's whereabouts did not. The parents reported that Max seemed to have appointed himself family guardian, alerting his parents to real and imagined dangers around the house, such as smoke alarms that might need new batteries, unlocked doors, windows left ajar, or a pot that might be too close to the edge of the counter. His sisters were beginning to tire of Max's fears of being kidnapped as they walked home from school. His mother, too, began to worry about perverts lurking in the bushes, so she armed the children with a cellular phone, which they carried to and from school.

In the initial hour of the consultation Max appeared "jumpy." He tried to play, but noises from the street or the hallway constantly distracted him. The chipped paint on a toy truck or a small tear in a doll's dress left him so preoccupied that he could barely set the stage for his characters, let alone begin to tell a story. About Billy, Max was blasé. Billy was in jail, and that was that.

Max's externalization did not effectively ease his anxiety. Even though he imagined Billy to be safely in jail, the anxieties that Billy's attack stirred now surrounded him. Danger lurked everywhere, and he had apparently lost the capacity to keep track of his mother.

If we focus primarily on Max's externalization as arising from his assessment that the world can and does pose real threats to unsuspecting little boys, we might be particularly concerned with the ways in which the abuse disrupted Max's previously established capacities, leading to a substantial impairment in reality testing. From this perspective, Max's need for attention to external events, quite understandably heightened following Billy's assault, appears to have become inappropriately generalized. Alternatively, if we were particularly attuned to Max's concern about external dangers as a representation of the fragility of his internal object world, we might assume that the abuse had undermined the stability of the internalized, soothing objects that previously enabled Max to move through life as an easy-going, affectionate child. From that vantage point, it appears that because Max can no longer locate his mother within himself, he must turn his attention to tracking his mother's movements in the external world.

The stories that abused children have to tell often gradually unfold into tales far more complex than they initially appear to be. Because physical or sexual abuse has such inordinate explanatory power in understanding the symptoms a child presents, they both impose great demands on the processes of evaluation and treatment. Even skilled and seasoned clinicians can easily be distracted by the known effects of abuse and thus miss important information that the child, through his symptoms, conveys. This may partly explain what happened in the initial therapeutic work with Max. The therapist appears to have been caught up in the parents' very moving and understandable concerns about Billy's abuse of Max. In joining them in their externalization, she missed the opportunity to explore the concerns that Max was expressing.

The story began one Sunday morning when Max, on the way to church with his parents and two sisters, had suddenly blurted out, "I don't want to touch Billy's penis anymore!"

His entire family was stunned by this dramatic announcement. Billy was a young college student whom they had met through church. Billy's family lived a considerable distance away and, with their minister's encouragement, Max's parents had taken Billy under their wing, frequently inviting him for dinner or on family outings. Fortuitously, just about the time their baby-sitter quit, Billy's work schedule began to interfere with his studies. Because Billy knew the children well, it seemed natural for him to step in. He easily took over their after-school and early evening care.

The parents had recounted the events of that morning many, many times. They had told the story to the police, their friends, attorneys, the first therapist and now again to the second therapist. He was struck with both how little relief the telling and retelling brought them and how little variation there was in their recitations.

As the parents described the scene that ensued following Max's announcement, they grew increasingly distressed. Just as she had in the car that morning, his mother burst into tears and continued sobbing as his father, with increasing anger, described bounding into the church, grabbing Billy by the collar, and being restrained by the other parishioners lest he "kill him." He concluded his story with, "They knew I'd do it, too."

During this scene, Max and his sisters sat in the car, the motor still running, with their mother still sobbing. Eventually, someone realized that the children must be terrified and drove them home while the minister and other members of the congregation dealt with the father, Billy, and the police.

The mother talked freely about her terrible sadness during the next few weeks and her acute fear of leaving Max with anyone, even previously trusted family members. She missed a great deal of work and described sitting for long periods, cuddling Max and crying. She felt completely "undone" by Max's continued symptomatology and repeatedly praised him for telling her about Billy, reassured him that he was not bad, and declared that she loved him best of all.

The father described feeling that his anger at Billy only intensified as Max's symptoms continued. In addition to pursuing the lawsuit against Billy, he kept in regular contact with those involved with the case, wanting to ensure that Billy was getting no special treatment. He rallied support among church members to have Billy excluded from the congregation and proudly announced that the one idiot who suggested that maybe Billy needed help, too, quickly learned "not to open her mouth again!"

The therapist suggested an extended evaluation, explaining to the parents that he would need to meet with them several times to get a more detailed history. At that time he also asked permission to speak with Max's teacher and the previous therapist. Max's parents readily agreed to this plan and seemed relieved that their concerns were being taken seriously.

Over the next several weeks, the level of chaos in which Max lived became increasingly apparent. He frequently arrived 15 to 20 minutes late for appointments, and his mother was, on one occasion, 30 minutes late in picking him up. When the therapist insisted that he could not continue with the evaluation under these conditions, the parents suggested that they could minimize the confusion if they put the mother's secretary in charge of scheduling appointments. They explained that they were essentially living in two homes, simultaneously trying to sell the first while renovating the second. The family's belongings were scattered between the two homes. They assured the therapist that this did not pose a problem for Max or his sisters, since this was the third time they had done this, and the children were used to it. As soon as the first house was sold, they planned to buy another for renovation and resale. In each instance, they tried to find houses that were relatively close together so that the children could walk to either place after school.

The therapist who had seen them for crisis intervention had noted that, like Max, his parents seemed "scattered," but from their description, this disorganization had appeared to be directly related to the abuse. She had offered to continue to work with Max if his parents wished, but she had not been overly concerned, since the family appeared to have a good support system, and the family members had mobilized themselves on their child's behalf. Max's telling his story had seemed to be helping him to overcome some of his sense of vulnerability; she had seen his concerns about dangers around the house as a predictable reaction to the molestation as Max attempted to overcome his feelings of helplessness.

On the other hand, the counselor at Max's school felt that the family's disorganization was particularly alarming because the parents showed so little awareness of its effects on their children. Max had been enrolled in this school at the beginning of second grade, having spent the first half of kindergarten in another private school, and the second half of kindergarten and first grade in the neighborhood public school. After many mix-ups and much confused communication, the counselor, in desperation, had taken to calling the mother's secretary as a means of informing the family of field trips and school holidays, or to schedule parent–teacher conferences.

She reported that, prior to the abuse, Max had seemed a remarkably resilient child, relatively oblivious to his surroundings; it didn't seem to matter much to him if he was late for school or late being picked up at the end of the day. He seemed to rely on his sisters or baby-sitters to keep track of his schedule for him. Max was equally easy going with his peers, seemingly happy to join in any game or activity or to stay on the sidelines if not invited to play. As for teachers, initially Max had seemed to like them all. However, in recent months, his teacher reported, Max had become extremely anxious at any separation from her. She had taken to walking him to the playground at recess and waiting with him until his sisters met him for the afternoon walk home.

The current therapist grew increasingly frustrated in his attempts to address these issues with Max's parents, who were unable to divert their attention from Billy and toward Max's internal world. His mother tearfully focused on Max's symptoms, wanting to know when they would disappear. She moved everyone with her profound sadness at the loss of the little boy who had seemed to progress through life with such ease and now saw danger lurking behind every corner. She longed for the previous closeness of their relationship, in which she felt that she and Max were especially attuned. Now she didn't know when he might erupt or how to comfort him. She felt that because of Billy she had lost her little boy. The father's concerns were different. He focused not so much on the actual assault on Max, but on how Billy's actions had betrayed his trust, generosity, and the good will he had extended to this young man. His primary concern lay in making certain that Billy was punished as severely and lastingly as possible. His story always began with Max's surprising announcement, which seemed to him the organizing event, the moment in which his trust in Billy had been shattered.

The therapist was never able to complete the evaluation. Max's parents could not reliably bring him to his appointments. Via a phone message from the mother's secretary, the parents indicated that business matters and the demands of managing two households made it too difficult for them to continue. Some months later, Max's mother phoned the therapist to say that she would call to set up an appointment "in a few weeks," but she never did.

Obviously, this case presents many complex issues, but for the moment, I want to consider the ways in which attention to external danger and the absence of a soothing internal object interrelate in the powerful maintenance of an external focus. Initially, it looks as if both Max's reality testing and the stability of his internal object world had been significantly disrupted by Billy's assault. However, on further reflection, quite an opposite hypothesis presents itself. The molestation, to which Billy actually confessed, certainly was disruptive, but rather than impinging upon Max's capacity for reality testing, it seems to have alerted him to the fact that his external world had for some time been permeated by dangers, dangers against which his typical detachment formed a poor defense. Max had protected himself against the chaos in schedule and surroundings by behaving as if everything were fine. Since he never knew for sure where or when he might find his toys, or himself, he became oblivious to his surroundings, making do with whatever presented itself. His apparently easy-going, affectionate relationships gave him the appearance of a child living in a world peopled by stable internal objects, whose continuous and comforting presence allowed him to make use of external objects to satisfy his needs. In actuality, Max did not form relationships, he simply and indiscriminately adapted himself to whatever children or adults presented themselves to him. In essence, he was a spacy little kid who managed reasonably well as long as the children, teachers, baby-sitters, or neighbors provided a benign environment.

But these primitive attempts to cope failed when something really bad happened to him. At that point his defensive structure could no longer protect him adequately against overwhelming affect. In the absence of stable internal objects, he was compelled to look to the external world for comfort and support. However, his parents made themselves no more available after the molestation than before; he really had not been safe, he had merely adapted to his parents' message that a life of confusion, chaos, and unpredictability constituted a perfectly acceptable state of affairs.

Of course, sadly and paradoxically, if Max's parents had been able to attend to his, or, for that matter, their own, internal world, the chaos of Max's environment would have greatly diminished. He would have internalized stable object relationships, which might have helped him withstand the disruptive affects following the molestation. So, from this perspective, Max's reality testing seems to be just fine. He is actually not worried about Billy—he knows where he is and that Billy no longer poses a threat. However, he can't keep track of his parents and correctly assesses that they are unable to protect him from danger. While we can understand the defensive posture in Max's suddenly assuming responsibility for smoke alarms or unlocked doors, we must also respect his belated recognition that his parents have created a world of such confusion and preoccupation that they might well not take adequate care to protect him.

We can readily understand Max's parents' wish to keep the attention focused on Billy and the molestation as the cause of Max's problems. Billy really did hurt their child. His behavior really did cause this little boy and the entire family enormous pain. And, despite their focus on Billy's actions, they really did hold themselves responsible for the molestation; after all, it was they who had befriended Billy. Superficially, it is also not difficult to understand why they would want to address Max's behavior as symptomatic of sexual abuse rather than as symptomatic of a disturbance in the parent–child relationship. And, because of Max's particular adaptations, they would have trouble comprehending that his symptoms stemmed not just from the moles-tation, but from his having no stable internal objects. The chaos they created around them externalized their own confused inner worlds. While they quite literally could not hold still for any therapy that relied on quiet reflection, their focus on capturing and punishing the "bad guy" did provide some relief and bring some organization to their affective turbulence. In situations like this, external reality can and does too readily provide demons, persecutors, abusers, and betrayers whose behavior offers explanations for, and allows for the focus of attention away from, sometimes equally or even more terrifying internal states.

In addition to confusion between inner and outer, externalization can also lead to a substitution of past dangers for future concerns. Certainly prudence dictates our educating children about how to identify and avoid potentially dangerous situations or people, but an overly zealous preoccupation with preventing child abuse may sometimes thinly disguise the projection of a past abuse into the future. Of course, the attempt to manage the feelings about what has already happened by attending to what *might* happen is doomed to failure.

Maria

Eight-year-old Maria was brought to treatment following her complaint that her paternal aunt "touched her" in a way that made her uncomfortable. Her plight clearly illustrates the dangerous consequences of externalization. The incident occurred when the aunt was helping both her daughter and Maria dry themselves after a bath. Maria's mother was distraught and enraged; much of her rage was directed at her husband for not having protected his children against his sister. The aunt was flabbergasted and intensely hurt by the vehemence of her sister-in-law's response. She insisted that she had merely cuddled her niece as she had many times before, totally unaware that it caused Maria any discomfort. She explained that she certainly would have stopped immediately had she known it was upsetting.

In the initial interview Maria's mother informed the therapist that she had been sexually molested during her childhood. She refused to elaborate, except to indicate vaguely that the perpetrator had been male. She explained that she had been too disturbed by the abuse to remember or discuss it. Over the course of the evaluation, the parents revealed the extent to which this abuse controlled the family's life. The children were never allowed to be away from their parents except to attend school. In the last year, Maria's father had suggested that, inasmuch as they were getting older, the children might be safe in the care of trusted relatives. Mother had reluctantly agreed that they could visit certain homes for short periods, as long as a female relative was present.

This mother's identity had become structured around the sexual abuse she had suffered as a child but about which she could not speak as an adult. She saw potential abusers on every virtually every corner and did everything within her power to protect her children from the external dangers that haunted her. She was unaware of the extent to which they, as a result, saw themselves as victims, even though, with the exception of the incident described above, there had been no reports of sexual abuse. In her attempt to maintain the externalization, the mother had assumed that, like the man who had accosted her, all perpetrators were male. Thus, even though her daughter had complained about having been molested by a woman, the mother sought a female therapist and never hesitated leaving her daughter alone in the room with the therapist.

Obviously, Maria's mother's constant vigilance toward potential abusers stemmed from a failure to resolve the abusive events in her own childhood. In her ostensible efforts to protect her children against potential future abuse, she actually made them prisoners of her own past. None of them was truly able to live in the present, that is, to create or reflect on his or her internal life. Maria's therapist noted that Maria exhibited astoundingly concrete thinking. Her most frequent comment was that she "didn't really have anything to say," except to report on events at home or school. Her capacity for fantasy appeared to be confined to persecutory fears about the viciousness of neighborhood dogs, prowlers who lurked around school and home, and the inadequate supervision of the playground at school. Indeed, in their efforts to keep Maria and her siblings in a safe environment, her parents had enrolled them in a small school, run by a family friend. However, the school's finances were so marginal that it was housed in a rather unsafe neighborhood and relied totally on parent volunteers for lunchroom and playground supervision. Children were routinely injured and bullied during recess; often they stayed inside to avoid encounters with the frightening people who wandered near the school.

Here we see the long-term consequences of child abuse that has not been integrated but maintained purely as an externalized danger. Maria's mother's judgment had been impaired by her identification of herself as a victim of sexual molestation, flawing her capacity to assess external danger accurately. Her behavior with her children suggested that she neither carried within her a reliable protective object, nor provided one for her children. Apparently having been unprotected from an external assault, she identified her continued anxiety as reality-based and as springing from the many dangers around her. She could not accept that she, like every other parent, simply could not protect her children from all possible dangers. Unfortunately, because she could not distinguish inner dangers from outer, past from present, she unconsciously pulled her children into her own world of projected persecutory fantasies, while she simultaneously placed them in potentially dangerous situations. Her behavior with her children repeatedly demonstrated her own profound sense of helplessness, both in the face of external dangers and in the absence of a soothing internal object.

The therapist felt that Maria could not turn inward, for in doing so she would confront a profound sense of emptiness. The aunt's touch that had alarmed Maria and her mother, rather than disrupting a stable world of internal objects, appeared to have offered Maria an identificatory bridge to her mother's world of external dangers. In therapy Maria had little to say about her aunt's touch, other than that it made her "uncomfortable." However, her sense of discomfort stimulated much discussion between mother and daughter as they attempted to negotiate the parameters of continued involvement with the extended family. Her mother routinely asked whether Maria should be kept away from her paternal relatives because of her feeling ill at ease. Periodically her father would, very tentatively, suggest that perhaps his sister really hadn't meant to fondle or frighten Maria. His questions about whether Maria and her aunt might discuss this event incited his wife's rage but seemed, over time, to give Maria permission gradually to lessen her assessment of how hard it would be to rejoin the activities of the extended family.

Her father's stance and Maria's increasingly clear statements that she really missed her relatives, who, after all, had constituted virtually the family's only social contacts, made it appear inevitable that Maria and her mother would again attend family gatherings. Once it was agreed that Maria would attend a favored cousin's birthday party several weeks hence, her mother turned her attention to ascertaining that Maria would feel completely comfortable leaving the party if she wanted, making sure that no one would be angry if she left with Maria, and gaining assurances from the relatives that she and Maria would be seated near an exit. The psychological inadequacy of these strategies became increasingly apparent as, over the weeks of preparation, Maria and her mother steadily added pounds and bulk to their already robust frames. The therapist, feeling that both mother and daughter were unconsciously turning to food for comfort and excessive weight for protection, tactfully voiced her concern that this young girl was quite rapidly becoming obese. The mother agreed that Maria had gained some weight but did not seem particularly concerned.

Within a few weeks after the birthday party, Maria's family members had resumed their usual relationships with the extended family. Maria's mother's complaints about feeling coerced by her husband continued, as did her monitoring of Maria's level of "discomfort." For her part, Maria, apparently feeling her additional padding offered her sufficient protection against external dangers, appeared happy to be reunited with her relatives.

These vignettes illustrate some of the many defensive strategies children employ in the service of maintaining an external focus as they attempt to prevent abuse from destroying the integrity of the non-abused self. With the exception of Max, who, prior to the abusive incident, appeared to make his way through the world in a state of rather benign dissociation, the children in the above examples did not rely heavily on dissociative defenses. Sam managed to maintain a relatively stable internal object through a kind of splitting that involved actually separating himself, as best he could, from interpersonal contact with the wrathful father, whose behavior threatened to weaken or destroy the internalized image of a loving, protective father. While these defensive maneuvers interfered with Sam's capacity to develop and hold an ambivalently loved object, they did allow for relatively cohesive representations of self and object. Sam simply created a "good" father and a "bad" father, which mirrored his interactions with his own father.

While Susan's mother was quite unpredictable in her temperament and behavior, her father was actually a relatively protective and stable object. Like Susan, he had learned to read his wife's moods, though with much more sophistication than his young daughter. With the help of her psychiatrist, he could actually buffer Susan against her mother's most malignant behavior. Sometimes he worked at home or hired a sitter; at other times he sent Susan to stay with nearby relatives; at still other times, he arranged for or agreed to psychiatric hospitalization for his wife. So Susan's highly developed attentiveness to her mother's moods served, in great measure, as an identification with her reliable, protective father. She could view her mother from the vantage point that a stable, internalized object allows. Because of the ongoing relationship with her father, continually supporting the soothing internal object world, she was able to withstand the threat of and actual abuse from her mother without the disintegration of self and object representations. This is not to suggest that Susan escaped unharmed or that she did not feel intense anger at and disappointment in her father, but that she, because of this relationship, was able to maintain and hold cohesive, ambivalently cathected self and object representations.

Like her mother's, Maria's world seemed almost devoid of internal objects. Maria presented herself as a victim of sexual molestation, but had so little to say about the abusive event that it was difficult to determine the extent to which her assertion of abuse was an accurate description of an event that caused her subjective discomfort, an identification with her mother as a victim of sexual abuse, an attempt to build an affective bridge to her mother, or an unconscious collusion with her mother's contention that the world is fraught with sexual dangers (Birch, 1998). In any event, the affective experience did not evoke a fragmented, dissociative state in Maria; rather it propelled her in the direction of a paranoid organization, in which forbidden thoughts and impulses could be well contained in the external world.

Particularly in the period immediately following the awareness or suspicion of child abuse, there is profound pressure to focus on the external—"What happened?", "Where did it hurt?", "How did it happen?", "Did it really happen?" In addition to turning attention away from the child's internal experience, questions such as these not only focus on the behavior of the perpetrator, but locate the abuse in the past rather than in the ongoing structuring of the child's psychic life. If we persist in this line of inquiry, we suggest to the child that our primary interest is in her ability to describe something outside herself rather than her response to that experience.

This attention to outward phenomena relies on the language of fact, action, and behavior. It suggests that an accurate historical account of the events is not only important but possible. However, as clinicians, our interest should be in helping the child manage the horrible, complex, and often conflicting feelings that come from abuse. These internal experiences are often not easily containable in words. The construction of an integrated, internalized story requires time and space for quiet reflection.

Chapter Seven

The Paradox of Language in Treating the Unspeakable

The ambiguities and hesitation that show themselves when children attempt to put abuse into language result not simply from linguistic immaturity or confusion, but from the particular meaning language has in the process of experiencing, internalizing, and knowing abuse. Many difficulties attend the task of putting language to abuse—but one that may go unrecognized is that the therapist must sometimes recognize and tolerate the child's contention that utterly no words can name or hold the internal chaos that inevitably emerges in the wake of abuse. The therapist, who typically values the organizing and liberating functions of language, is powerfully tempted to name too quickly what the child finds to be unnamable. Paradoxically, when we put language to an experience that the child either cannot name or has deliberately, whether consciously or unconsciously, endured by separating it from linguistic formulation, we necessarily to some extent falsify the child's experience and run the risk of subverting the treatment. Before language can successfully be brought to treatment, the therapist is obligated to recognize and withstand the wordless, chaotic terror in which abused children live.

Professionals who work with abused children often disagree about whether these young victims can talk about what happened to them. Certainly, some children do actually report abusive events and can do so without prompting by adults. Abused children are neither mute nor incapable of conveying their experiences. However, we must distinguish between children's descriptions of external events and their narrations of internal experiences.

Even young children may be able to give a reasonably clear and accurate account of another's behavior, such as, "He touched my pee-pee"; nevertheless, this information may belie the child's affective and cognitive confusion. A child's verbal report of physical or sexual abuse relies on the ordering function of language in describing experience. However, a relatively organized narration about behavior may sometimes deflect our attention from the disarray of an internal world. Partly because behavior is observable and feelings are more difficult to discern, the former is easier for a child to describe. Thus, the ordering function of language illustrates a paradox confronting those of us who try to understand the world of abused children. If we too quickly attempt to impose the organizational powers of language or too readily accept the child's ordered and reasonable descriptions of abuse as the whole story, we may collude with the child's defensive use of language to mask the more troubling and less accessible feelings and cognitive confusion. We may very well desire to accept a child's straightforward narrative as evidence that she has internalized and resolved the abusive experiences she describes. Indeed, children are often encouraged to bring order to these experiences so that those who have harmed them can be stopped. However, in a psychoanalytic treatment, where the external demands for order are removed, the falseness of this structure often shows itself quite quickly.

The narrative structure evident in clinical work with children who come to treatment from a background absent of abuse frequently stands in striking contrast to the fragmentation and confusion that can and often does permeate the therapeutic sessions of abused children. Because of their different relationship to language, children who have not been abused are far more likely to engage the therapist in a mutually created story, whereas abused children often demand a rigidity in the therapeutic relationship and process. Even in their chaos, abused children must maintain control over the therapy; they allow little to chance and do not easily tolerate the therapist's introduction of modifications or variations in words or play.

Just as we have come to appreciate the importance of narrative structure in the development of a cohesive sense of self, we have come to see psychotherapy as a creative process. This joint endeavor engages both patient and therapist in the development of a unique story (Hewitt, 1993; Ogden, 1997) that describes and expands the possible outcomes. However, the propensity for action common to children in therapy often adds a dimension that transforms the therapist's office from a quiet sitting room to a stage in which the child's unfolding drama engages patient and therapist. So despite the importance of narrative in psychoanalytic work with adults, it often plays a relatively minor part in successful therapeutic work with children, for whom action is so crucial.

Of course, no one can create a paradigm that can successfully contain all of the possible variations children present in therapy. As a way of conceptualizing the intertwining of behavior and commentary that characterizes psychoanalytic work with children, I would like to discuss a continuum of therapeutic communication that ranges from the largely narrative at one pole to almost pure action at the other. Although the concepts of pure narrative without action or simple action without intended communication are illusory, they offer useful theoretical endpoints on a continuum. Somewhere in the space between narration and action, most of child therapy takes place and might be conceptualized as a therapeutic theater. The child straddles the roles of playwright, director, and actor in his efforts to demonstrate, as well as describe, his compelling internal dramas. This continuum only superficially concerns speaking and doing; more important, it is about the relationship between patient and therapist, the child's desires and capacities to be known, and the therapist's ability and willingness to participate in the unfolding of the child's unconscious processes.

At one end of the continuum, we find those therapies that are largely narrative, where words contain and convey action: patient and therapist talk, listen, and reflect together; impulses and activities are as frequently described as enacted. This occurs exceedingly rarely in therapeutic work with children—and virtually never in the initial work with the child who has been abused. Even if the abused child sits quietly and talks, there is seldom enough trust or comfort for reflection.

The patient who can rely on words alone to convey her thoughts and feelings demonstrates a willingness to entrust her story to the imagination of the listener. The desire to be known by another, not just as presented, but as reflected in the vision of the self created in the mind of the other, requires a rather remarkable capacity for trust.

Those who have been deliberately ill-treated simply have no access to such faith. Without the reliable and repeated experience of a cohesive self in relation to another, one person cannot simply and straightforwardly tell another about one's self. Thus, the child who has relied on the fragmentation of dissociation to endure repeated beatings or sexual molestation does not have a coherent, cohesive story to tell.*

A psychotherapy conducted largely within a narrative structure depends significantly on spoken language with its power to order and organize. For example, rather than arrive late, an adult patient might begin an hour with the comment, "I was so mad at you that I thought about coming late today." In this statement the patient indicates his awareness of his affective state and the possibility of action for expressing that state. However, he made a conscious choice, at least in this instance, to talk about rather than act on his feeling. Perhaps this choice had something to do with the patient's wish to communicate his anger clearly to his therapist rather than allowing any ambiguity. But action (particularly in psychotherapy, which relies so heavily on clarity of motivation and meaning) is often much more ambiguous than words. Suppose our angry patient had elected instead to act on his feelings and come late to his appointment. While waiting, his therapist would have time to reflect on any number of possibilities for his patient's absence, including his being caught in traffic, or staying away in an effort to avoid uncomfortable feelings, or either consciously or unconsciously attempting to invoke certain feelings in the therapist. The actions are ambiguous. Not until he arrives for his appointment can the patient and his therapist begin to talk together, to use language to create a shared understanding of the meaning of and motivations for the actions.

A narrator feels more or less content to tell his story, but the playwright has determined that her tale must be *shown* as well as told. She creates a cast of characters; she scripts their words and choreographs their movements to evoke the changing visual and auditory images that she wants the audience to hear and see. In the context of

---

*This does not mean that the child will be unable to give a relatively straightforward account of the facts surrounding the abusive events. It sometimes is the case that children either because of developmental immaturity or defensive confusion cannot relay the "facts of the case." However, if the internal experience has been chaotic, confused, and fragmented, then a coherent narrative falsifies, rather than describes that experience.

the narration–action continuum, we should recall that when rehearsals finally begin, the early practices are typically devoted to "blocking," that is, to mapping out the movements that will carry the actors from one scene to the next through the acts that eventually compose the whole. Relationships and unconscious motives are graphically demonstrated by physical movements. The attuned therapist pays careful attention to the child's movements as well as to the direct and indirect instructions the child gives her. As in the case of Amy (see Chapter 4), who offered the therapist a doll as a means of bringing her closer, children's directions are often nonverbal. In other instances, children explicitly engage their therapists as actors in elaboration of their internal dramas with detailed verbal directions.

Joey

As 5-year-old Joey settles into a therapy session in front of the dollhouse, he hands me the mother doll; articulating script and stage directions, he informs me how I should play my part.

"She comes home and says, 'This house is a mess!'" instructs Joey.

With the help of the more junior dolls, Joey then gleefully wreaks havoc upon the dollhouse and its contents. On cue, I march the mother doll into the chaos, announcing, "This house is a mess!"

Finding me an inadequate actor in his drama, Joey sighs scornfully, "Not like that."

As he takes over the operation and voice of the mother doll, he relegates me to audience. At least for the moment, he has determined that I am incapable of accurately enacting the drama he has in mind.

Joey's "firing" me bears further consideration. He clearly wants me to know his feelings, but at that instant, for whatever reason, he cannot coach me until my performance meets his expectation. To convey successfully what he envisions, he has essentially two choices—to tell or to show. He does not move toward a narrative description of the scene he imagines with a comment like, "No. She's madder than that," or "You should sound more sad"; instead, he shifts into action in order to demonstrate.

Sometimes, as teachers and parents well know, demonstration works far more efficiently than description, particularly if the language available to the teller or listener cannot sufficiently circumscribe the complexity of the image or action to be conveyed. For example, consider trying to teach a child to tie his shoes without any reliance on demonstration! Even worse, try to imagine having to learn this complex series of twists and turns from narrative description alone.

We make an extremely important assumption that operates when we tell, rather than show, our stories to another—an assumption I believe we take too much for granted. The willingness to trust in the imagination of the other, to allow ourselves and our stories to be created in the mind of another, can, it seems to me, come only out of the conscious or unconscious conviction that the integrity of the self-as-presented will not be destroyed. When we narrate ourselves and our histories, we expect that what develops in the mind's eye of the reader or listener will approximate closely enough the setting, the characters, and the action we wish to convey. Sometimes patients, as Joey did, need to determine whether their trust in the therapist's imagination is justified. Others, perhaps more certain of their skills as raconteurs or with more positive experiences of being benignly held in the mind of another, feel more willing to proceed without feedback, to act on faith, even when that faith is not well placed.

Barbara

Over the course of a lengthy treatment of a young woman named Barbara, I developed a very clear picture of her mother. Since Barbara's relationship with her mother supplied a primary focus of our work together, I had a significant amount of information about the mother, a rather tall, large-boned, blond woman. I had ideas about her friends and knew that she dressed in bold colors and often spoke in a booming voice. Over time, in my mind's eye, I could easily see Barbara's mother moving through the house in which she raised her family and hear the conversations my patient described to me. In essence, I developed a comfortable familiarity with her mother's character and image; I felt that I had come to know her well.

In the context of termination, Barbara described browsing through old photo albums. She commented, "In looking at the pictures of my mother, I was struck again by how much you look like her! And you sound alike, too. You're both so soft-spoken." I was stunned, confused, and annoyed. As I attempted to fit this tall, blond, strong-voiced mother into my self-image as a small, dark-haired, soft-spoken therapist, I felt as if I had just seen a remake of a favorite movie, in which the previously familiar heroine had become almost unrecognizable!

Because Barbara had entrusted her reality to my imagination, her narrative had permitted me the countertransference privacy of creating a fantasy of a larger-than-life mother, quite different from me. Our exploration of the collusion that allowed me to maintain this distorted image of her mother made up an important final piece of our work.

In the context of the narration–action continuum, I want to emphasize that precisely because Barbara did not demand that I describe my visual image of her mother, I was enabled to build from her narration an autonomous fantasy of a mother who could protect us both through her transference storms. Unlike Joey, Barbara did not need to check to see if I was getting it right, nor correct my assumption upon discovering that I hadn't. She could tolerate not needing to know exactly what I was thinking. While my fantasy of her mother did not at all fit external reality, it did accurately reflect Barbara's wish for a strong, sure, and protective mother, one who could tolerate her outbursts without either crumbling or resorting to sadistic retaliation.

I believe that as Barbara shifted between her views of me as either excessively rigid and mean or, alternatively, weak and ineffectual, I must have conveyed in many ways that I had created an image that approximated, closely enough, her wish for a mother who was strong and powerful without being cruel.

In retrospect, a number of factors influenced Barbara's willingness to undertake the process of therapy largely from the position of narrator. She was bright and had a significant command of language. While difficult and not without trauma, her childhood had not included abuse. Perhaps most important, although far from perfect, her relationships had been sufficiently stable and benign for her to develop some faith in the good intentions of others.

Unlike Barbara's therapy, the therapeutic work with abused children begins at the far end of the continuum from narration in the world of action, action often lacking apparent meaning. Listening to these children can prove exceptionally difficult because they are often trying desperately to believe that what they have to say did not happen, is not real, and does not matter at all. The very events that propelled them into treatment often comprise what they most want to deny, negate, or at least minimize. Putting words to these events gives them form and substance—creates meaning and ownership. But that is precisely what abused children are so often mightily trying to avoid. And so they are left without a language to know or share their experiences.

Children who have been physically or emotionally abused exist in the world of action, not merely because the structure of language is developmentally, neurologically, or defensively unavailable, but because narrative structure has been destroyed as a means of psychic survival. If an experience is truly crazy, as abuse is, then it defies the child's attempts to contain it in the orderly, rational world of language. The abused child cannot think or speak or act sensibly precisely because her story makes no sense. This leaves us with a powerful paradigm that may be particular to therapeutic work with abused children: namely, the destructive function of language in the treatment of something unspeakable.

We repeatedly encounter the idea that abuse is unspeakable. It is unspeakable because the horrific facts are felt as a shameful secret. It is unspeakable because there are no words to capture events that shatter the child's capacity to integrate experiences. But beyond these and more dreadful than these, it is not speakable because the very fact of putting language to an inherently disruptive experience falsifies that experience.

Paradoxically, this means that to hear what abused children have to say requires being able to listen to their actions without interpreting meaning where none exists. Of course, actions do sometimes have meaning and are used as both conscious and unconscious forms of communication. However, for many abused children, the actions are intended to destroy meaning, to prevent the development of a coherent story.

I do not mean to imply that abused children literally cannot use words; indeed, often they can quite articulately describe abusive events to police officers, attorneys, or therapists. Alternatively, their quick-witted verbal attacks on those who try to help them provide clear evidence that they understand the power of spoken language. Instead, I mean to suggest that, perhaps out of our reluctance to truly know the horrors they wish us to understand, we are often powerfully tempted to focus too much attention on these words as conveyers of meaning and to respond with verbal interpretations. In doing so, we may unwittingly help abused children to create a fundamentally untrue narrative, a facade of cohesiveness and pseudomeaning that merely masks the underlying chaos. So when the children resist our attempts to talk, to name, or to organize, we might understand their protests not only, for example, as a defense against overwhelming affect or a resistance in the service of protecting the image of an idealized parent, but as a plaintive cry that we are not really listening to the story they need to illuminate. If, instead of talking, we listen, not just to the content of their words but to the process of their language—the ways they use speech to connect with us, deflect our attention, inform us, or hide from us we may learn what *they* want us to know.

Louise

Louise was about 10 when she was referred by her school because of her lack of friends, difficulties in accepting any kind of criticism, and horribly disruptive outbursts of temper. When her parents first came to meet with me, I was struck with her mother's rage at the school. Her diatribes would permit no questioning or disagreement. She found her daughter virtually perfect in all ways and believed all difficulties were either caused by the school or resulted from their faulty perceptions. Nevertheless, largely because she felt coerced by the school, she elected to have her daughter begin treatment with me.

Louise was a bright, articulate child but far from charming. A pattern emerged very quickly in the therapy hours: Louise routinely gathered several puppets, which she gave unusual and difficult-to-pronounce names. Then, fast and furiously, she would charge through a story in which the character thought to be good was discovered to be bad, or the mother was really the daughter, or the cousin had come disguised as some other character. At first I tried to make sense of the names and to follow the content of the changes, assuming that going from bad to good, for example, might have meaning. The characters exchanged rapid-fire comments, often followed by Louise's eerie cackles. I usually couldn't keep the stories straight, but when I tried to clarify my confusion, my questions were typically characterized as stupid.

During this time, Louise's mother came in for one of our regularly scheduled visits. She began her usual tirade of complaints, but I was astounded to hear that her vicious attacks were now directed at Louise. She described Louise exactly as the school had done, only in far crueler terms. She proclaimed that she certainly could understand why the teachers and students hated this child, who was abhorrent in every way. Everything the school complained about could be attributed to Louise's shortcomings or her incorrect perceptions.

Although I had no reason to believe that Louise or her sisters had been physically harmed, the unrelenting viciousness of her mother's diatribes certainly constituted verbal abuse. I now understood the hours with Louise as repetitious illustrations of the unpredictability of her world, both inner and outer. Just as the content of her mother's verbal attacks had to be warded off, Louise used spoken language not to convey the specific meaning of the words, but as props in a confusing, erratic drama. The words, like the names that I could barely understand, let alone remember, were intended to disguise, not reveal. The rapid movement from one character to another, from one affective state to another had as its purpose blocking out the words that were too painful and difficult to hear. Louise could not tell me in a straightforward narrative what it felt like to be with her mother. My understanding of the meaning of her play required that I temporarily move away from language, relinquish my effort to analyze the content of her play. Before I could help her put words to her experiences, I had to allow myself to absorb the fear and confusion that permeated her life at home and ripped through the hours with me.

We have all experienced frustrating moments in which we recognize the inadequacies of language. We attempt to describe a dream, a daydream, a tender moment, or our responses to a work of art, and in the very moment of doing so, we feel the experience slip away from our very efforts to capture it in language. Sometimes we respond angrily, feeling that our words have failed us, other times with sadness that we cannot use language to make a connection to those we want to tell about ourselves, or we respond with resignation and defeat, feeling that the story can never be truly told.

Usually we accept and adapt to the limitations inherent in transforming primary process experiences into the linearity of secondary process thought. That is, we make meaning as best we can in order to capture and convey the experience. However, the essential difference between these experiences and the experiences of the abused child is that the child has no desire to capture the abusive experiences or little interest in conveying to us the horrors that brought her to our attention. To do so, for her, is to make meaning of something that does not make any sense at all. In my experience these children have a powerful wish to retain the abusive experience as fragmentary, elusive, unnamable, and unnamed in the mistaken belief that doing so will reduce the power of the experience and maintain it in the external world. For better or for worse, once we can name a thing, we own it, and it has a place in our internal world.

A young woman who had repeatedly been abused during her childhood described her reluctance to discuss or know anything about the perpetrator of the abuse.

> "I don't want to think for even one half of one second about him, about why he did what he did or even about what he did. That would mean it might make sense. Even thinking about it, having a thought, thoughts come in words, if I can even think it, that he might have had a motive, that he thought about it, then maybe it was something I could understand. Understand? Understand what? How could I understand it? It cannot be understood."

We can comprehend the confusion between understanding and condoning or forgiving. But that is not what this young woman was talking about. Her worries were more basic, they derived from the terror of seeing a coherent picture in the fragmentary confusion of memory and fantasy, with the terror of thinking, lest she give form to something she desperately wanted to relegate to the world of shapeless nonreality.

In the aftermath of abuse, children live in a dark, eerily kaleidoscopic inner world, in which organized images and thoughts can be punctured without warning by fragmented pictures, flashes, sounds, and feelings. An adult patient who had been abused as a child frequently talks of her terror of sleep because of the dreams of abuse. These dreams contain no coherent pictures, no scenes of what was done to her; rather, they are fragmented, disjointed images that fade and flash, one permeated by another, until she wakens in terror and exhaustion. "But," she sighs, "it's no different when I'm awake."

Michelle

The disorganization in which abused children reside was aptly demonstrated in the treatment of a 6-year-old girl who was hospitalized following her attempt to jump from a second-story window. This child's physical abuse at her mother's hands was well documented; sexual abuse was merely suspected. Regularly and in myriad ways, Michelle forced her chaotic, enraged neediness upon her therapist. During many sessions she could barely maintain self-control, either virtually or actually hitting, kicking, or lunging for toys to throw or break. Her wails and moaning cries echoed through the hallways. Repetitive, relatively organized play could, at any moment and without apparent provocation turn to primitive, incoherent shouts and invectives. In one session, her therapist's announcement of a 2-week vacation prompted 20 minutes of uninterrupted, ear-piercing screaming, which culminated in her vomiting on the office floor. Her therapist left the session in a state of physical and emotional exhaustion born of her having to restrain Michelle while posing to herself the inevitable questions about whether the crying represented an expression of emotional pain or whether she might be suffering from enormous physical pain as well; whether the child would ever stop; whether she should try some other means to stop her; what her colleagues in neighboring offices must be thinking; what she could have done differently; and how she would ever present this hour in supervision. Perhaps Michelle's vomiting was an intentional communication; perhaps it just served to culminate too much crying and too much misery. In any event, it brought the hour to a dramatic close.

Even though Michelle appeared to function at higher levels of ego organization at times, the sudden emergence of primitive states did not appear regressive. Indeed, although the primitive images of neediness, greed, rage, and terror did not always loom at the forefront of Michelle's daily internal life, they always appeared to coexist with states of greater ego organization. It was as if Michelle's psychic "house" contained two adjoining rooms—one organized, the other in disarray. Sometimes she lived in one and sometimes in the other.

This, in fact, appears to be one of the frequent psychological characteristics of victims of child abuse: The movement in and out of primitive states is lateral rather than vertical; that is, the shifts do not involve a regression; Michelle's more primitive behavior did not result from defensive regression, nor did it emerge as a consequence of the safety of the therapeutic environment. It just formed a part of Michelle's story.

Michelle's first session following her discharge from the hospital tells her story well. She began, as she often did, by cooking. This time she made cocoa.

"You're the baby," she said. Looking at an imaginary watch, she continued, "If you're late I'm gonna whup you. You have to take off your shirt, your shoes," pointing to all the pieces of clothing her therapist was supposed to remove. The therapist asked, "You're gonna whup me naked?"

"Unh-huh, in the bath. You're gonna take a bath and then I'm gonna whup you and hold your head in the water until you drown."

Ignoring the therapist's questions about this, Michelle lay on the floor and proclaimed, "You're the doctor. Get your bag. I'm dead."

"What happened?"

"A boy raped me—on Saturday morning—in the park."

"What happened?"

"On my back, with a raper. He hit me."

"What's a raper?"

"Like a grass raper, what they rape grass with," she replied pointing to her back. "He killed me and now I'm a robot and I'm running out of batteries."

"Do you want any battery juice?"

"Yes, now I'm coming back to life, listen to my heart."

"Is it a little girl's heart?"

"No, it's a robot heart. I'm a robot. Bring back the robot girls. Not the boys. The boys are bad. Just girls. I'll protect the girls. Now I'm a baby." She put a toy bottle in her mouth and crawled into the lap of her therapist, who was feeling quite overwhelmed by this flood.

The therapist commented, "Every baby needs a bottle."

"Mama. Mama."

"Yes, you have a mama and a grandmother."

Michelle instantly became a dog and began angrily stuffing the pieces of the tea set, in which she had earlier served cocoa, into her greedy mouth.

I believe it would be a mistake to focus on the content of this hour, to assume that any single story led to another or that the content of the material gave rise to intrusive anxiety leading to what looks like, but is not, a play disruption. There is very little play to disrupt;

rather there are a series of images, some of which appear to be more coherent than others. This session occurred very early in the treatment, and the therapist did get caught in attending too much to the content, as, for example, when she assumed that Michelle was trying to tell her in words about being molested.

What matters in this session is that Michelle became disorganized by her experiences of abuse and neglect, and she brought that disorganization to the therapy. I believe Michelle simply acted out the chaos of her internal world, a world in which images do not hold still and words have little meaning. If we assume that Michelle offered these snippets as a deliberate although unconscious means of connection, we would undermine the actual communication emanating from Michelle's actions. Unlike Joey, Michelle cannot control what pours forth, and when her therapist doesn't quite understand, Michelle's language does little good in redirecting the action. In other words, Michelle, at this point in her therapy, cannot assume the role of either playwright or narrator—she lacks access to the interrelated structures of language and observing ego that would allow her to describe her inner experiences and to shape her therapist's behavior by verbal cues or direction.

Michelle's uncontrollable wailing at the announcement of her therapist's vacation differs in degree, though not in kind, from normative episodes familiar to parents of young children who are just beginning to master language. For example, Johnny has awakened happily from a nap. His mother, anticipating his hungry state, takes him to the kitchen for a snack. When he brushes aside the cookie she offers, she asks what he would like. He answers, "Cookie." His mother briefly offers the original cookie again; then, since Johnny is quickly becoming increasingly agitated, offers, in quick succession, other varieties of cookies and crackers. Johnny pushes them all away, wailing, "Cookie." Finally, stalling for time, his mother pours a cup of milk. Johnny calms and happily downs the milk along with the original cookie.

Though this brief vignette offers many possible avenues of discussion, I use it here to illustrate a normative occurrence of children's inability to turn reliably to language as a means of structuring and describing an affective experience. Michelle's loss of language is frequent, unpredictable, and not easily recovered. In contrast, Johnny's difficulty in finding words emerges in a period of regression, as he struggles to fully awaken. Developmentally, Johnny has not achieved sufficient command of language for us to consider its absence a loss. It is a capacity in the process of developing—sometimes available and sometimes not. What does Johnny mean by "cookie"? Has he condensed "milk and cookie" into one word? Perhaps, although his mother responds as if they have a shared understanding of the word "cookie." His mother's actions, I believe, convey a much more profound understanding of Johnny's repeated, distressed, wailing of "cookie." She offers a number of alternatives, finally shifting to a different category of food. She responds as if Johnny has said, "I'm feeling really miserable right now and what I'm saying isn't working to get what I want, but I don't know what else to say." Ignoring the literal definition, she takes Johnny's word as an affective communication, *including that he has no appropriate words to convey his intended meaning.*

We should also note Michelle's "rape/rake" confusion in this context, because it reminds us how easily children confuse words, meanings, and affects. Was Michelle raped or was she raked? Maybe neither; maybe both. The facts of what happened in the park may well be unknowable to both Michelle and her therapist, but the affect that overwhelms a cohesive story line is almost palpable. Michelle's therapist does want to understand her, does want to listen to the story she has to tell, but like Louise's tale, Michelle's story has embedded itself in a swirl of primitive, overwhelming affects.

As therapists, who appreciate the power of language, we want to help these children create a history out of the fragmented chaos of abuse that repeatedly and unexpectedly threatens to intrude. We want them to have stories that they can hold without terror, stories that do not inundate them with overwhelming affect. We can do this effectively only when we can, with them, repeatedly endure the affective disorganization that eludes language. Although we use words, initially, our patient attention and our affective steadiness are far more important than what we say in helping these children settle into a calm, alert state in which their feelings are experienced as signals and we are experienced as benign, even potentially helpful, people.

Only after we tolerate the world of action without meaning can we begin, with the child, to build a vocabulary for actions, feelings, and relationships. If we too quickly name, interpret, or describe a child's experiences, we merely offer children a false narrative—one that distances them and us from the truth of their experiences. When we keep ourselves outside the child's world, our words serve only the purpose of shielding ourselves from the horrors they need us to know.

Chapter Eight

Good Guys and Bad Guys: The Temptations of Splitting

People who abuse little children are bad guys; those who help them are good guys. If the world could be divided so easily and neatly, our clinical work with abused children would be much easier and more straightforward. Out of a conscious wish to spare the child additional pain, we would like to slam the therapist's door in the face of the bad guys. Despicable people; we don't want them in the room with us! The temptation for therapist and child to divide the world into "good guys" and "bad guys" can be quite powerful, especially when we feel pressured by external forces to clearly separate the two—to assign guilt to the perpetrator and thereby, assure the child of her innocence.

In this very delicate arena, it is essential that the therapist remain absolutely clear about the distinctions between moral, legal, and psychological issues. No matter how sexually, emotionally, or physically provocative they have been, children cannot be held responsible for instigating their abuse. It is the moral obligation of the adults in the child's environment to maintain the boundaries between child and grown-up and to exercise control of their impulses. Legal determinants of guilt and innocence are complex and are not the province of psychotherapists. We must focus exclusively on the child's psychological experiences of good and bad, guilt and innocence if we are to most effective. It is in this arena that the two often come together in ways that makes us uncomfortable.

No matter how much we might condemn an adult who has abused a child, we must assume a neutral stance toward the child's internal representation of the abuser. This does not mean that we assume a morally neutral position. It does mean that we keep ourselves open and equally receptive to all of what a child has to tell us about herself, her experiences, and her representations of her abuser(s).

If we reassure her about her innocence when she feels guilty, she will not believe us and, worse, will surmise that we do not understand her. If we set ourselves the task of educating her about how to protect herself in the future, she will assume that she should have been able to do so in the past—and that she shares in the responsibility for her abuse (see Chapter 5). If we offer an abused child our patient attention, we will come to know, with sometimes overwhelming intimacy, how it feels to be the "bad guy" and how it feels to be his victim. Given the intense discomfort these primitive feelings stir in us, we should not wonder at finding ourselves often tempted to discover ways around truly apprehending the mind of the child. No matter how much we would like to keep the "bad guys" out of the therapy, they will inevitably make themselves known through the affective interplay between child and therapist.

Psychotherapy with abused children is not an easy endeavor. These children do not trust easily; they test our patience over and over again. They fear their own impulses and ours; they attempt to provoke our loss of control in manifold ways. They think they're crazy; we begin to feel crazy when we're with them. They feel damaged; we wonder if they are beyond help.

In our initial meetings with the child, we may learn directly, or only through subtle hints, about the dreadfully painful thoughts, feelings, and experiences that will emerge over the course of an extended psychotherapy. This knowledge may, more frequently than we would like to admit, quietly contribute to the recommendation for brief therapy or crisis intervention. We may support this suggestion by emphasizing factors in the child's psychological status (such as lack of language) or factors in the environment (such as the level of disorganization) that will make it hard to sustain an ongoing, reflective psychotherapy. We may conclude that a psychotherapy that depends on reflection, or learning about intrapsychic processes through the examination of interpersonal exchanges, may be just *too* hard, even impossible.

However, if child and therapist *can* embark on a course of psychoanalytic treatment, the complexity of ideas and feelings surrounding the abuse will be woven into their ongoing interchanges. While it may take time for the patterns and nuances unique to this particular therapeutic pair to emerge, there are common paradigms in the work with abused children that may show themselves relatively early in the therapy.

Rescue fantasies can easily be enacted in the treatment of any child, but they may be particularly compelling for those working with children who have been dreadfully mistreated (Gillman, 1992; Cohen, 1988). In this paradigm, child and therapist collude in the profound wish that the therapist will quickly and easily deliver the child from the misery that seems to beset him at every corner. The following vignette illustrates how this fantasy can play itself out with people trying to help a desperate child. Their demands that the therapist "*do something*" often intensify when their attempts to save the child have either come to naught or repeatedly have been dashed by the child's seemingly willful misbehavior.

Marcus

People often commented on Marcus's striking features; his almost unearthly beauty and uncanny charm drew people to him in quite remarkable ways. From preschool through third grade, Marcus had attended a private school that had originated in the era and spirit of the counterculture of the 1960s. While initially an exciting, experimental school, after a few years, it had lost most of its luster and good standing. However, it did continue to draw students from a small cluster of parents who wanted a free and unstructured program for their children. Unfortunately, Marcus's mother, who lived in a state of disorganized psychotic anxiety, was unable to maintain any vigilance over Marcus's home or school activities. So, even after one of the teachers was fired because of inappropriately sexualized behavior toward the children, she continued to use him as a baby-sitter for her son. Marcus began protesting having to spend time with this young man; his mother became convinced that Marcus had been sexually assaulted. Without warning, one afternoon she packed all of their belongings, fled across the country, and enrolled Marcus in the most staid school she could find.

The school quickly discovered that Marcus's skills were far below grade level. Like others before her, the student teacher in his class found Marcus almost irresistibly charming and volunteered to tutor him after school. This lasted a few weeks until one day, when she asked Marcus to try a new assignment, he registered his protest by throwing his chair across the room.

This prompted a recommendation for psychotherapy along with a referral to a more experienced tutor. She too was charmed by Marcus. His sad history and the ongoing plight of having to live with his mother's psychosis only endeared him more to her. The new tutor assured the therapist that the student teacher merely had not had enough experience to work with Marcus and, given that he had no obvious learning disabilities, that he could relatively easily be brought up to grade-level work.

Things went smoothly for several weeks. Pleased with her success, the tutor suggested that perhaps others simply had not understood Marcus very well. Indeed, the tutor and Marcus had settled into a seemingly comfortable relationship. One day she presented Marcus with an assignment that was harder than usual. He resisted, but the tutor, confident that Marcus could handle the work, persisted with her expectations. In response Marcus spat in her face, tore up his book, flung it across the room, and knocked over his desk as he stormed from the room.

This outburst understandably hurt and dismayed Marcus's tutor who, unfortunately, refused to continue with him until his psychological problems were "settled." After a lengthy conversation, the very real hurt behind the tutor's thinly veiled criticism of the therapist became apparent. She had expected her relationship with Marcus to be different; he had initially responded to her care, which only fortified her sense of being the one special person who would get through to this child. However, Marcus's inability to withstand any narcissistic vulnerability completely prevented him from allowing closeness or tolerating even a hint of failure. He made others fail instead.

The tutor was neither the first nor the last of well-intentioned people who tried and failed to rescue Marcus. Many factors prompted these attempts. People responded to his physical beauty and superficial charm; they knew the strains his mother's mental state placed on him and felt sorry for him because of his troubled past. They did not realize that Marcus, like many children with similar backgrounds, could not tolerate any closeness in a relationship. Intimacy terrified rather than sustained him. When faced with the possibility of failure, he could not turn to another for comfort or assistance—that would expose an unbearable need for help. And, because Marcus had not had the kind of relationships that had allowed him to establish reliable, sustaining internal images, he could not turn inward for comfort. Thus, the moments in which he anticipated failure put him in an untenable psychological position. He responded to the people who were trying to help as if they were enemies, threatening to expose his frailty and vulnerability.

With great frequency, we find the important people in the life of an abused child divided into two feuding camps. Often, one group seems to stand for protecting the child, feeling that the other group treats the child too harshly or makes too many demands on a child who has already suffered greatly. The second group often seems to stand for setting reasonable, but firm, expectations, feeling that the child's bids for comfort or leniency are simply attempts to use the hurt she has suffered to manipulate others into meeting her demands.

These divisions among the people around an abused child reflect the split in the child's world of internalized relationships. Because of the actual overwhelmingly bad people in the child's life, his internal world consists of "good guys" and "bad guys." Even when these children cognitively appreciate that most people are neither all good nor all bad, affectively, it is very difficult for them to sustain positive images of people in the face of disappointment, anger, or hurt. In the aftermath of abuse, children have trouble developing and maintaining the capacity for ambivalently held relationships. Thus, if someone they like or love hurts or angers them, that person becomes "bad." Affectively, this is a very different experience from feeling angry, hurt, or disappointed in someone we like or love; we retain our positive image of that person even in the face of negative feelings. For an abused child, negative feelings, which are often cataclysmic affective experiences, destroy the positive images. From this vantage point, we can see why these children often feel so bereft and so utterly alone.

A facet of human relationships that underlies psychoanalytic psychotherapy is our proclivity for repeating or evoking aspects of past relationships in current ones. Pushed by powerful forces, we repeatedly create relationships that match those in our world of internalized images. If we expect to be treated well, we will find caring, respectful people and/or tend to evoke those feelings in those around us. If we expect ill treatment, we will find it, provoke it, or see it, even when it isn't present, in the feelings and behavior of others.* Obviously, abused children have every reason to expect ill treatment and, because of the enormity of their own negative feelings, they have the power to provoke intense feelings in others.

Sometimes, children who have been abused successfully and repeatedly provoke those around them into harsh or even abusive behavior. Until the child's world of internal figures contains more benign images, therapists, attorneys, teachers, or social workers can be drawn into an unending, futile battle to protect the child from continued mistreatment. For example, a child who has been sexually abused is taken into protective custody. When his first foster parent hits him, he is moved to another home. In the second placement, his behavior so outrages the foster parents that they insist on his quick, unplanned removal. In the group home where he goes next, he so brashly and repeatedly breaks the rules that his counselor's efforts to discipline him begin to verge on the sadistic.

The vignette below illustrates the strong influence an abused child can have on her own environment. Ruby's behavior fueled a battle between school and home that graphically depicts both splitting and the intensity of feeling that a troubled child can evoke in those responsible for her care.

Ruby

Dr. Brown had been seeing 7-year-old Ruby only a short time when he received a call, resonating between pleading and rage, from the principal at her school. The principal insisted that Dr. Brown come in for a conference as soon as possible; Ruby was out of control, her foster mother belligerent, and her social worker unavailable. Dr. Brown agreed that Ruby could be very taxing but wondered if anything in

---

*This is a very rudimentary outline of "transference," which in all interactions, including the therapeutic relationship, is highly complex and nuanced. For example, we evoke feelings in others that we don't expect, as well as those we do; we incorrectly, as well as corrctly, interpret the behavior and responses of others; and those with whom we interact contribute their own histories, expectations, and interpretations to the relationship.

particular had prompted the principal's sense of urgency. The principal, a veteran teacher, relatively new to school administration, described her enormous sympathy for Ruby and the horror that she had endured. Her concern had prompted her repeatedly to intervene with teachers and children on Ruby's behalf. When Ruby became disruptive in the classroom, she had offered her the opportunity to come to the office to "help" the secretaries until she could calm down. Ruby seemed to like this distraction, but it had little effect on her classroom behavior. The principal had then decided that, rather than helping Ruby, this program was instead rewarding and reinforcing Ruby's misbehavior. As an alternative, she wanted to consider brief suspensions from school, hoping they might be more effective. However, according to the principal, the foster mother (who was in fact, Ruby's aunt) not only had no interest in coming to the school to remove this unruly child, but had angrily suggested that the principal was just trying to cover up the teacher's incompetence by "dumping" the school's problem on her.

Not unexpectedly, the foster mother, or "Auntie," had a somewhat different view of the situation. She felt that the principal was woefully naive and far too untried to take on the challenges of this particular school. She experienced the principal's requests for help alternately as "whining" and the result of a racial bias, which, to her way of thinking, placed too high a premium on very controlled behavior. She was not the least bit interested in this principal's sending Ruby home in the middle of the day!

Auntie had only reluctantly taken on the responsibilities of foster parent to her niece. The matriarch of a large extended family, she had, in addition to raising her own children, acted as temporary or substitute parent for many children over the years. However, when approached by Ruby's social worker, her genuine fondness for this little girl, along with a deeply held conviction that children belonged with family, had made it impossible for Auntie to refuse the responsibilities of being her foster parent.

From the beginning of her contact with Dr. Brown, Ruby's aunt had spoken openly about feeling "too old and too tired" to manage this very troubled little girl. Despite this characterization of herself, she was a spirited woman who commanded a great deal of respect from family and friends. She knew too much about life in the housing projects to hold an unrealistic optimism about Ruby's chances for recovery and escape.

Ruby had gone to Auntie's following her discharge from the

hospital. She had arrived at the hospital in a catatonic state, having been severely beaten and thrown down the stairs of her home, ostensibly as punishment for helping herself to a soft drink belonging to her mother's boyfriend. Because of the mother's long and extensive drug use, the court determined that Ruby should remain in protective custody following her release from the hospital. Ruby's Auntie was well known within Children's Protective Services as an experienced foster parent with a no-nonsense approach to raising children. What she lacked in warmth, she made up for in steadfastness, even in the face of the most aggressive and difficult behavior.

At school, Ruby was a little terror, routinely sent to the principal's office for behavior that petrified her classmates. She moved about the classroom whenever she pleased and aggressively intruded on other children's studies. She frequently threatened to and sometimes actually did throw a chair at children when she didn't like what they said or did. At home, where there was less stimulation, Ruby exhibited more contained behavior. However, even there she suffered enormous anxiety; she anxiously rubbed her head until she created bald spots and was frequently overcome by seemingly unprovoked crying spells. Neighborhood children's understandable fear of her allowed Ruby to win at most games and to commandeer the toys or treats she wanted. Once, shortly after a child refused to give Ruby the candy she wanted, she stole it and bloodied the child's nose in the process.

In contrast to her behavior at school and at home, Ruby approached her therapy with Dr. Brown as a model citizen. She spoke only when spoken to and played with toys only when they were offered to her. Dr. Brown was particularly struck by her carefully controlled one- or two-word responses to all of his questions or comments, especially in light of her apparently total lack of impulse control in other settings. She never protested going to therapy; in fact, her foster mother reported that she looked forward to the sessions. Yet she played with excessive control and without joy.

After a few sessions, Dr. Brown voiced his observation that she was particularly quiet whenever she came to therapy. Ruby responded, "You get in trouble at school if you talk out of turn." Silently wishing that Ruby's misbehavior were that minor, Dr. Brown explained that therapy was not like school and that she was free to talk whenever she wanted, adding that he, in fact, would be very interested in anything and everything she had to say. Ruby seemed to take this in, and over the next few weeks, she began to display more openness in both her play and verbal interactions.

In this context, then, Dr. Brown was ordered to appear for a school conference. He and Ruby were just beginning to know each other. Although he had some hunches about what might lie behind Ruby's controlled demeanor in the therapy sessions, his ideas were still untested hypotheses, yet to be explored with his thus far exceedingly well-behaved patient. Perhaps Ruby wanted to demonstrate how well she could "follow the rules" in order to win his love or to avoid his anticipated wrath, or both. Perhaps, also, in the quiet of the therapy sessions, Ruby's despair, otherwise hidden behind her aggressive attacks, showed itself. And perhaps she just didn't have any words to say what was in her mind, or else what was in her mind was not in words, so that she was, in fact, showing the pervasive emptiness that emanated when she felt the need to exercise strict control of her thoughts and actions.

If Ruby hoped that Dr. Brown would rescue her, she wasn't saying so directly. However, the principal, having failed in her attempts to save Ruby from herself, was certainly asking to be rescued by somebody.

As a skilled and experienced clinician, Dr. Brown had few illusions that Ruby's behavior could be transformed as quickly or as completely as her teachers, classmates, or principal might wish. Her first 7 years had been marred by neglect and abuse; she was a child fighting for her life with no very good reason to trust that others would act in her best interests and every reason to anticipate a brutal attack at any time from any corner. Like so many children whose stories of neglect and abuse engender an outpouring of sympathy from those who hear them, Ruby was more appealing when considered from a distance. The day-to-day reality of trying to teach, or discipline, or play with her quickly turned sympathetic responses to fury, helplessness, and hopelessness.

Not surprisingly, Ruby's world quickly divided itself into "good" and "bad" objects. The principal and foster mother found themselves at odds, each seeing herself as doing the best possible job under extremely trying circumstances, while viewing the other as incompetent and difficult. Indeed, the conference confirmed Dr. Brown's suspicion that, through the complex interplay of conscious and unconscious forces that swirl around an abused child, these two women, with Ruby's help, had actually succeeded in getting each other to behave as badly as they were accused of doing. Dr. Brown saw his task as attempting to bring ambivalence back into what had become a dangerously polarized object world. Without it, the adults responsible for

Ruby's care had lost their capacity to appreciate each other's efforts and accept their own inevitable mistakes. If one has placed all of one's unacceptable hatred and loathing into another, one cannot then allow oneself to feel as the other must. The empathic failure that pervaded the relationship between Ruby's home and school seemed to have grown, at least in part, from each woman's reluctance to accept how much she truly loathed this child.

Dr. Brown's clear and unabashed statement that Ruby often made it hard for people to like her temporarily opened the way for a discussion about the problems Ruby created for those trying to help her. Auntie and principal could each grudgingly admit at least to the other's good intentions on Ruby's behalf, but Ruby's show of mean-spirited defiance quickly closed the door on any chance of an ongoing discussion between home and school. Dr. Brown resigned himself to fielding periodic enraged calls from one woman or the other until Ruby could be moved to a new school. There, Ruby again successfully created a split between home and school, but without the racial undertones to fuel the flames, the situation did not become as bitter or decisive.

Although Ruby often treated others quite badly, she had the good fortune to have an "Auntie" who did not mistreat her, even though she often felt like giving her a smack or two. In this case, the split between home and school may have actually protected Ruby from the full wrath of either her aunt or her principal; they could direct their anger toward each other rather than at Ruby. At least temporarily, their fight also may have served to keep Ruby's provocative behavior out of the therapeutic relationship.

When a child can successfully, even though unconsciously, split her world into good and bad figures, the therapist may feel strongly compelled to align himself with those who show sympathy toward the child. He may find himself forgiving the child for even the most unconscionable behavior or rationalizing that her ill temper or misbehavior must stem from continued provocation or a lack of care and understanding. When carefully examined, we often discover that these are means to avoid the knowledge that we don't like this child any better than those who complain about the outrageous nature of her behavior. When she successfully provokes people to mistreat her, our harsh criticism of them, though well-deserved, may also mask the extent and intensity of the negative feelings she stirs in us.

An abused child's capacity to stir in us the most passionate hatreds (Schaer, 1994; Birch, 1994; Chused, 1991), not toward the abuser, but toward the child herself, certainly ranks among the most difficult aspects of therapeutic work with abused children. It promotes our participation in splitting, as we look toward external reality for the "bad guys." If we can find them outside of the therapeutic relationship, we can continue the fond, but futile, hope that we will not have to confront them in ourselves. We would like to prevent our entering into the inevitable reenactment of the abusive relationship. However, only by allowing ourselves to accept the various roles the child assigns us will we come to know the fullness of her experiences.

We are relatively familiar with the rage, helplessness, loathing, or impulse to retaliate that abused children can stir in their caregivers and therapists. Equally painful and maddening is a state absent of feeling. However, since many abused children exist in a state of psychic numbness, we would reasonably expect that, if we can tolerate it, they will use the therapeutic relationship as Peggy did, to demonstrate this profound sense of emptiness.

Peggy

Eight-year-old Peggy was referred for treatment following the discovery that she and two other children had been sexually molested by Alex, a 14-year-old boy, at a recreation center they all frequented after school. When the full extent of the abuse came to light, the director of the center expressed doubtful surprise, wondering how the children could have been out of her sight long enough for the events they described to have occurred.

The director had interviewed each of the children, as had the police and an attorney hired by one of the other parents. Believing that participation in the investigation would give Peggy a sense of power, her parents initially supported the interviews. However, when Peggy began to develop increasingly elaborate justification for not telling an adult about the molestation, they became concerned that the questions seemed to focus too much on whether the director could or should have discovered the abuse and on the efforts the children had made to alert adults.

All of this happened within a few days. By the time Peggy reached therapy, she was mightily tired of talking about "this mess." The repeated questioning, particularly about why she had not told anyone, had left her feeling guilty and disappointed in herself. She also felt extremely sad, confused, angry, and anxious. In the first therapy session, she confessed that she knew she should have told "right away." All along she had planned to trap Alex, but now she understood that she should not have tried to take care of things herself because she was "just a little kid and little kids aren't supposed to have to take care of things."

Peggy's plans for an elaborate entrapment had been a means of trying to protect herself from fear and humiliation during the abusive episodes. Inadvertently, the repeated, well-intended, reassurances she received following the discovery of the abuse undermined Peggy's, albeit misplaced, confidence that she could manage on her own. By praising her for talking, the interviewers contributed to Peggy's guilt over *not* talking sooner. The reassurance that she should not have felt responsible for stopping Alex sometimes made her feel that her plans had been "stupid." At other times, she insisted that she just hadn't explained her strategies well enough and that they really would have worked. So, while the cessation of Alex's molestation of these children can only be viewed as positive, the investigative process and the meanings Peggy made of it became an integral part of the abusive experience and heightened its negative impact.

In the beginning of treatment, Peggy offered a brief description of some of the abuse, though she insisted on leaving out some of the details because they were "too gross" or required using words that she didn't want to say. I commented that she must be pretty tired of talking about all of this, but that I would be happy to listen to what she did have to say about Alex, what had happened at the recreation center, or anything else she might want to talk about.

Peggy's greatest interest lay in telling me about her plans to catch and expose Alex. Tentatively, she began to describe some of the plans she had devised. Since I was genuinely interested in how this little girl had understood Alex's overtures, her compliance with his demands, and her subsequent imagined defiance of his power over her, I listened attentively as she told and retold the plots and subplots. When I expressed sympathy for how hard it could be for a child to think clearly and creatively when feeling very frightened or worried, Peggy declared that I wasn't understanding how good her plans really had been. She decided to draw pictures of the hideout so she could demonstrate her plans to trick Alex and show the director what he was doing.

My assigned task was to figure out the plans by looking at the drawings. No matter how I tried, there always seemed to be a clue I missed. When I asked about a particular element of the drawing, Peggy frequently chastised me, "I told you that already."

Sometimes she declared that a tiny peephole was hidden in her drawing of the hideout. I had to find it. Peggy assured me that it was "really, really easy to see," unless, of course, you are "really, really stupid." Not surprisingly, I routinely felt and was declared to be "really, really stupid." Sometimes the peepholes were no bigger than a dot left by a pencil tip; sometimes Peggy chided me for being so ridiculous that I couldn't even tell that the holes were "invisible."

Over the course of the hours in which Peggy drew, I made a number of observations about our interactions. Sometimes I noted that as long as I had only really, really tiny clues we could still hope that if I had bigger clues I might be able to learn some of what Peggy wanted me to know. Other times, I spoke about how scary it was for children when adults weren't paying enough attention to keep them out of danger. Sometimes I suggested that, even though it didn't make her feel very good, it might seem better to think that I was stupid about little things than stupid about big and important things. At times Peggy tolerated my direct comments about our interactions, but sometimes she could bear only comments containing more psychological distance. When she could tolerate a connection with me, she might respond by giving more information or allowing me to participate in an elaboration of the drawing. When she too strongly feared my disappointing her, she might simply offer no verbal response or tell me to "shut up."

In the sessions in which the manifest content concerned Peggy's attempts to trap Alex or secretly reveal the molestation to her teachers, Peggy was often quite talkative. Although her narratives were choppy and harder to follow as her anxiety increased, she did try to communicate verbally. A typical description of her plot to trap Alex might go something like, "I put some stuff up there and then over the table, but then it didn't go, so we—well, and then on the floor. A tent. A tent with a hole so you could see. You could see in, too. You could, really. The kids were *real* noisy. Teachers don't hear too good when kids are noisy." This chatter might be interspersed with requests for a crayon, a question about whether I had seen her favorite TV show, or a quick, startled query about a noise she heard in the hallway. Peggy imbued these sessions in which she tried to communicate to me about her efforts to act on her own behalf with lively energy.

When Peggy was feeling particularly vulnerable, she frequently came to her sessions armed with one of her many illustrated books of drawing lessons, which followed a sort of line-by-line approach to drawing. Her affect in these sessions was often a pressured, good-natured, pseudofriendliness as she carefully demonstrated her ability to follow the directions precisely. Indeed, her figures, which she drew again and again, appeared to be almost identical to those in the books. Any trace of spontaneity, individuality, or genuine affective connectedness effectively disappeared into generic illustrations.

In these sessions, the rules that I had to follow were as exacting as those the books dictated to Peggy. I could comment on how well she followed directions, how hard she worked at the drawings, or how important it was to know that she could make these pictures exactly right. Now and then I might be allowed, without an interruption from Peggy, to say something about how the pictures in the book were very helpful in showing some things and hiding others. Typically, in sessions dominated by the drawing lessons, Peggy simply began talking over me if my comments veered too close to the psychological.

However, my own drawing was permissible. In contrast to other sessions or with other children, at these times with Peggy, I did not proceed with spontaneous drawings; rather, I began with a lesson from her book, but tried to introduce into my drawing some variation, more or less, depending on how frightened she seemed. I assumed that these books, in part, offered a statement about her terror at the possibility of becoming overwhelmed by the emergence of unconscious material. By starting from one of these absolutely predictable drawings and gradually introducing new or different elements, I hoped to indicate that together we might find a way of taking small steps toward discovering what so frightened her.

My suggesting variations on the theme also represented a way of trying to avoid succumbing to the internal dangers of these excruciatingly boring sessions. When I allowed myself to consider the meaning of Peggy's behavior, I couldn't help knowing how successfully these books put a wall between us, as well as any affective connection Peggy might make with her own internal world. The books quite specifically concerned *not knowing*—putting aside one's own ideas or images and following the dictates of another.

Sometimes the pressure to keep still felt almost overpowering. I wanted to break the silence, to share my insights with Peggy, to make a connection with her and relieve my sense of being locked away with my own thoughts. As I made myself wait for those moments when I thought perhaps Peggy could listen to what I had to say, I came to understand the oppressive dread Peggy must have experienced in waiting for just the right moment to trap Alex.

Not knowing when I might find an opening, I waited. Wondering whether my comment would be scornfully cast aside, I waited. Pondering the validity of my wish to speak about my own unease, I waited. Desperate to break the cheerful, unyielding silence, I waited.

I recognized my sense of impending doom in the sessions when Peggy smilingly approached with her drawing books in hand. I dreaded those hours, and I did not like Peggy at all during those sessions. I had come to know how tenuous my emotional survival seemed in these sessions. When I allowed myself to reflect on the process of the hour, I became acutely aware of being trapped with my own thoughts, of feeling utterly alone, unable to find a bridge to Peggy.

Sometimes my mind wandered and I would find myself daydreaming. These trivial diversions allowed no space for Peggy but provided an antidote to my feeling helplessly imprisoned in my own thoughts. Alternatively, when I forced myself to attend, to stay in the room with Peggy, a kind of deadness settled over me. She steadfastly chattered about the drawings, insisting on my admiration, but allowing no space for a genuine response from me.

When I recognized the banality of the daydreams I drifted into at these times, it occurred to me that their appeal for me paralleled the appeal the drawing books held for Peggy. Both were utterly devoid of meaning but seemed to offer a refuge from the life-and-death struggle Peggy brought to psychotherapy. Peggy used her drawings to eradicate meaning and I, in turn, mirrored her dissociated emptiness in my daydreams. In this way we were joined in a deadly nothingness of not thinking or feeling or knowing.

Like the little girl hiding in the tent trying to communicate through "invisible peepholes," when I could think, I was left alone with my own thoughts. Just as she had felt her knowledge was too dangerous for parents or teachers to hear, I sensed that Peggy felt my thoughts would be too dangerous for her to know. On the other hand, Peggy's quiet insistence on the pretense of a relationship required my emotional deadness as well as hers. We could behave as if our communication had importance or meaning, but, in fact, it just involved drawing the same affectively empty pictures over and over again.

In this vignette, we can see how Peggy's behavior effectively communicated her own state of psychic numbing and her sense of the impossibility of a vital understanding between us. Our being together depended on an affective deadness, which, paradoxically, meant that we had no meaningful relationship. However, if we could think together, then we risked having feelings so powerful and awful that they might destroy the relationship. It seemed that Peggy felt she had to settle for an empty relationship, lest her feelings destroy the vitality of a connection that allowed for thoughts, feelings, and genuine interaction.

I hoped that by tolerating the deadness Peggy imposed on me, I would eventually convey my willingness and capacity to bear with her the feelings she felt to be unbearable. When she could not stand my comments about her feelings, I tried to put my interpretations into actions, instead of words. For example, if I could change a drawing just a tiny bit without worry that I had ruined it, then perhaps Peggy could, as well. And if we could begin to look inside for images or ideas to introduce into our drawings, then perhaps we could begin to look inward at other thoughts and feelings. Through this process, I could gradually help Peggy put words to the thoughts and feelings that so frightened her and by doing so, help her limit their power over her.

Children who fight, spit, scream, swear, or physically attack their therapists are difficult indeed; our reluctance to walk into a session with them appears rather simple and straightforward. We see ourselves as helpers; they treat us as the enemy. Even as we try to control our rage and our wishes to fight back, we can take a somewhat empathic stance toward our responses. We even expect sympathy from colleagues or consultants.

Although children who have been abused do often overtly behave as if they want to kill us, sometimes their quiet attempts at "soul murder" are even more insidious and successful. When a child hits or shouts or fights, we can, with relative ease, view our wishes to retaliate as a response to the violence they attempt to inflict on us. No matter how difficult it may be, there is an affective connection.

However, when a child hides his terror and rage behind a smiling mask of superficial good humor, he prohibits an affectively vital relationship. In these situations, we run the risk of retraumatizing the child by our efforts to make contact. We are prone to risk rationalizing our attempts to enliven ourselves as being in the best interests of the child—after all, we are simply trying to make affective contact through our comments, or questions, or offers at play. Instead, our task with a child whose physical and emotional life has nearly been snuffed out is often first to endure the profound emptiness—to know with the child how it feels to be among the living dead.

Chapter Nine

Collaborative Work with Parents

Whether it is the parents or substitute parents who bring a child to psychotherapy, the caretakers of an abused child often arrive at our offices in a state of massive confusion. These children can be persuasive actors. Because of this they have often successfully, although unconsciously, convinced both those around them as well as themselves, of their ability to exercise control over their emotions and behavior. Rather than expose their feelings of helpless confusion or depression, they may manifest a variety of behavioral symptoms that effectively mask an underlying sense of profound vulnerability.

So while the child may not feel or act confused, those caring for him often do. Parents and foster parents complain of overwhelming feelings of helplessness and uncertainty. Their confusion may stem from their own lack of clarity about how best to help the child. However, their emotional state may also reflect the feelings the child carries within him, but cannot articulate. The child's capacity to transfer his feelings or evoke powerful affective responses in others, particularly in those closest to him must not be underestimated (see Chapter 8).

If the child has successfully externalized his internal chaos, then those around him may both feel and act chaotically or incoherently. His caretakers may feel that they just don't know how to help him—that nothing works. They may find a response that comforts him or helps him to control his behavior one day and is completely useless the next. Unfortunately, when the child's unconscious drama of helpless confusion draws adults into it, a cycle of blame and recrimination can quickly come to dominate child–caretaker interactions. Thus, the child, rather than consciously feeling beyond help, experiences potentially helpful adults as inept and utterly unable to find ways of easing his misery. At times these adults may accept this view of themselves; at other times, they may feel that the problem lies with the child—that he is a hopeless case. This perception may represent an unconscious identification with the child's view of himself as a person damaged beyond repair. We can easily imagine the wildly careening feelings and contradictory behavior that can result from these shared unconscious processes.

For these reasons, the therapist must pay careful attention, whether through observation or report, to the affective experiences of parents, foster parents, social workers, or teachers. To the extent that those responsible for the child's care have come to contain the child's unarticulated and unacceptable feelings, their complaints and concerns may provide the first window into the abused child's inner world. Particularly when abuse has led to provocative, uncontrolled, or violent behavior, the child's caregivers are understandably frightened about the child's safety and the well-being of other family members. They may also express concern about their own emotional lability in trying to live with this child, who routinely moves them from great sympathy to intense rage.

In other cases, parents or foster parents may describe feeling that they have "lost touch with" or "can't reach" a child, whose behavior is otherwise quite normal. This feeling of an unbridged emotional distance can cause pain and disorientation, particularly when the adults both want to and are genuinely trying to help. Obviously, the therapist may find herself in the same position—feeling unable to make a connection to the child, confirming everyone's belief that the child is "unreachable."

Equally dangerously, if the therapist does not attend to and work with the dynamics between herself and the parents or caregivers, she may be all too willing to accept the idealized role of the child's savior. This only increases the parents' sense of inadequacy and may ultimately lead to a disruption of the therapy. Sometimes children are moved through a series of therapists, with the complaint that the previous therapists simply weren't helpful or that the child never really made a connection. Clearly, this can occur, but sometimes it was the parent who failed to feel connected to the therapist and, feeling left out or inadequate, moved along in the hope of finding someone who could successfully collaborate with the parent's wishes to help this suffering child.

Successful and sane parenting requires a certain amount of denial. All parents know that, despite their best efforts, any child may be injured, killed, or struck by a crippling illness. However, unless stirred by news of a seriously ill child, an accidental injury, or a premature death, parents generally put this knowledge out of their minds, lest effective parenting become virtually impossible. This awareness may lead to anxiety of almost psychotic proportions, or, on the other hand, to the virtual smothering of a child's independence in order to preserve the illusion of parental omnipotence. When parents are confronted with the actuality or serious likelihood that their child has been abused, the knowledge shatters the normative illusion that they can keep their child safe.

The vicissitudes of parental responses to the discovery that their child has been abused have multiple determinants, including the particular characterological vulnerabilities people bring to parenthood as well as the meaning and circumstances of the abusive incident(s). For some parents, the loss of illusory omnipotence triggers an enraged response. Other parents, faced with the crumbling of their denial, confront the limitations of their capacities to protect their children with depression and helplessness. In either event, the child suffers; when the distressed parents are overcome with feeling, they are not fully emotionally available to their child.

The magnitude of this loss can overwhelm some parents leading to an actual breakdown in the ego functions that would enable them to help their child manage the physical and psychological sequelae of the abuse. Other parents can engage in the struggle with their own emotional responses without withdrawing from or overpowering the child who so desperately needs their attention. Even when parents do have the ego strength to muster their emotional resources on behalf of their child, this may be a temporary or intermittent state of affairs.

Amy

Amy's mother (see Chapter 3) is a good example of the fluctuation in a distressed parent's availability. When Amy's parents first suspected that her older playmate, Jeffrey, had been fondling her, conflicting feelings bombarded them. Jeffrey and his parents were friends of the family, which only intensified their worry and confusion. They wondered whether Jeffrey's behavior resulted from his having been molested, which they thought might allow them to feel some sympathy for him. They considered the possibility that the children had really just been engaging in "doctor play," which would not cause concern. They also thought about whether Amy's budding sexual explorations had influenced Jeffrey's behavior, and whether their child's early loss of innocence would leave her permanently scarred. Emotionally, they just couldn't seem to settle anywhere.

In the first session, Amy's mother guiltily confessed that in the days following their discovery of the suspected abuse, she was distracted by her preoccupation with these questions. Sometimes just looking at Amy caused her to burst into tears; Amy would then be worried and confused, which would, in turn, intensify her mother's guilt and grief. She described feeling terribly helpless and angry—angry at herself, Jeffrey, and his parents. While she knew these teary episodes only upset and confused Amy, she found herself unable to control her outbursts. Repeatedly, she described her guilt over making Amy endure her show of feeling.

Through careful exploration of the events that led Amy's parents to seek help, I was able to help the mother appreciate the very real and helpful actions she had taken on her daughter's behalf. She had comforted Amy, listened without prodding, tolerated Amy's regression, and altered her own schedule to accommodate Amy's greater need for closeness. As her awareness of her actual effectiveness as a parent increased, the mother could put her "crying jags" in perspective. Although she had indeed burst into tears on a number of occasions, she had also contained her fearfulness relatively quickly, using conversations with her husband and friends to protect Amy from the outpouring of her feelings. There was some basis for this mother's guilt over being unavailable to her child, but her emotional distance had been intermittent and transient.

Max

By comparison, Max (see Chapter 6) did not fare so well. His parents were so affected that they were unable to contain their affects and impulses, prohibiting them from functioning as effective parents. The mother became overwhelmingly depressed; her initial response of sitting, tearfully immobilized in the car while her husband went after Billy, barely diminished over time. She described cuddling and rocking Max, not so much to comfort her child, but to soothe and reassure herself. Unable to contain or manage her affective response, she was unable to mobilize herself into effective action on behalf of her child.

In contrast, Max's father, who was barely prevented from assaulting Billy, relied on action to ward off his feelings of depression and helplessness. Although his rage at the person who had molested his son is understandable, he, like Billy, lost control of his impulses. In doing so, he abdicated his responsibility to his child. At the moment of disclosure, Max needed his father's comforting attention. Instead, the father instantly and intensely focused on punishing the perpetrator. Unfortunately, over time, he continued to direct his attention toward Billy, and in the sessions with Max's therapist repeatedly expressed his dismay over Billy's betrayal of him and the goodwill he had extended to this young man. Although Max's father was sympathetic to his son's plight, the abuse constituted such an emotional assault for him that he could not differentiate his own hurts and needs from those of his young boy. In addition to the pain the father suffered on behalf of Max, Billy's abuse of this man's largess profoundly injured his self-esteem, his sense of his own good judgment, and his view of himself as a good and protective father.

The child, the parents, and potentially the larger community have much to gain when parents make concerted and thoughtful efforts to help identify or prosecute the person who has harmed their child. It is paramount, of course, and everyone hopes that the perpetrator may be prevented from hurting any other children. However, despite the importance of cooperation with police and attorneys, we must not overlook the extremely potent lure of external solutions for internal conflicts. While successfully prosecuting a child abuser may well instill or restore a sense of power in the victims and their parents, it also adds to the complexity of the psychological issues confronting the children, their parents, and the therapist.

Whatever problems prosecution solves, it cannot undo the crime. Like adults who contend with childhood sexual abuse, these children and parents intensely desire that the abused child be restored or recreated magically in a "pristine" condition. This wish that abuse could somehow be eradicated, that their history could be reversed, provides an important, though easily overlooked, motivation for a sometimes relentless search for "what really happened." The pursuit of the perpetrator surely constitutes an attempt to prevent further abuse; it can, however, also serve to rationalize the unconscious belief that if only he can be located and forced to confess, if there can simply be an accurate reconstruction of the crime, the original sin can somehow be undone or prevented.

For some parents, unrelenting guilt over their inability to prevent the abuse of their child or to recognize it earlier leaves them vulnerable to identifying themselves as profoundly inadequate, impotent parents. Ironically, if this sense of themselves becomes pervasive, their actions may actually begin to conform to their self-images as parents, thereby diminishing their capacity to provide adequate care and protection for their children. An insidious pattern easily develops in which the parent's sense of helplessness drives an unconscious need to prove that the abuse actually could not have been foreseen or prevented, that is, that her sensed helplessness has firm roots in reality. In an unconscious and powerfully dangerous attempt to reassure herself that actual protection was impossible, the parent may continually expose her child to situations of potential danger.

Therefore, it is imperative that the therapist work with parents to distinguish between their actual and perceived helplessness. As Amy's mother began to accept the significance and success of her efforts to help her daughter, her sense of impotence understandably began to diminish. Only then could she grapple with her sense of having ignored feelings of discomfort about the particular playmate who hurt her daughter. Initially, she countered her helplessness with a conviction that the boy had displayed clear signs of being a brutal and troubled child. She berated herself for ignoring what she *knew* to be true: that this boy was a child molester in the making whose parents showed woeful negligence in supervising their son. Gradually, as she could tolerate more ambiguity, she tempered this idea, leaving her with the awareness that she had felt vaguely uncomfortable about Jeffrey's behavior, though she could never precisely identify what in particular made her a "little nervous."

She could then also consider that she tended to worry more than her friends about her daughter's safety. In fact, she thought her friends' gentle teasing about her overprotective stance might have influenced her to allow Amy to play at Jeffrey's house, despite her concerns about his inadequate supervision.

As her first response to learning that her daughter had most likely been molested, she had intensified her previous hypervigilant stance, severely curtailing her activities so that Amy would never be out of her care. To a great extent this was a reasonable, empathic response to Amy's regression—a regression also fueled by the mother's anxious conviction that her lapse in attention led to Amy's having been molested.

Over a period of months, Amy's mother began to integrate a recognition of the extent and limits of her capacities to protect her child. She did have more "uncomfortable feelings" about situations than most of her friends, but in most instances, Amy emerged unharmed. Slowly she could become more precise about which externalities and internal processes gave rise to these discomforts. Then she could act accordingly. So when Amy was invited to a birthday party at the home of a child whose parents she didn't know well, she arranged to stay at the party. When she became anxious about Amy's going to the zoo with a dear friend of the family, whom she had known and loved for years, she recognized that her discomfort had to do with her own internal state. When she could recognize and accept her own sadness over Amy's budding independence, she could then allow her daughter the freedom to enjoy this outing.

Eventually she could, with enormous unhappiness, accept the part her own psychology had played in Amy's being molested. Both her overprotectiveness and a brief counterphobic foray into perceived external danger stemmed from her own concerns. She had attempted to manage her own intense separation anxiety by externalization, which then allowed her to rationalize keeping Amy close to her. Unfortunately, because her projections made so many things seem potentially dangerous, she could not reliably assess external danger. Furthermore, her awareness of her heightened sensitivity led her to discount the judgments she did make, feeling that her fears were "all in her mind," anyway.

Although Amy's mother brought many of her own fears to Amy's treatment, she was never confused about who had actually been injured. She did not forget that her anxieties, guilt, and self-doubt were either created or intensified by what had happened to her child, that is, that her own feelings were important, but secondary. For Amy's mother, the molestation was extremely upsetting, but not traumatic. It did not overwhelm her typical defensive strategies, nor did it massively interfere with her usual coping patterns.

Amy's mother initially approached me as the expert who would know better than she how to help her daughter. She asked for books to read on child development, abused children, and how to help children make friends. Amy's molestation had undermined, though not overwhelmed, her sense of herself as a good parent. Therefore, in this case, it was extremely important for me to eschew the role of the expert who had the most important knowledge about Amy. Indeed, Amy's mother knew far more about her daughter than I did. She needed help in recognizing and mastering the anxieties that interfered with her making her knowledge conscious and mobilizing the necessary judgment and resources on behalf of her child. Helping her to do so allowed for truly collaborative work, in which I, as Amy's therapist, could direct my efforts toward developing a shared understanding of the ways in which the abuse had disorganized the family's individual and collective representations of mother, father, child, and family.

Rebecca

In other cases, an abusive incident can lead to confusion, rather than disruption, of parent–child representations. Rebecca's parents brought her to treatment shortly after her entrance into first grade. Although she did not particularly enjoy kindergarten and had been described by her teacher as "touchy," she had completed the year with few absences and reasonably good relationships with teacher and peers. However, her anxieties about school grew over the summer holiday, reaching phobic proportions by the beginning of school. At first, her mother tried staying in the classroom briefly, but, rather than diminish Rebecca's need for her mother's presence, it seemed to increase her clinging and intensify her demands for her mother to remain. Her mother then arranged to help in the classroom for more extended periods, but Rebecca's anxieties still did not abate. When she refused to go to school on the days her mother did not work in the classroom, both her parents and her teachers felt that outside consultation was in order.

In the first session, Ms. D, Rebecca's mother described her confusion about how to understand and manage her daughter's fear of school. The time she had spent in the classroom sufficiently reassured her of the kindness and competence of the teachers. The children were also friendly; she observed no bully or any children whose lack of impulse control would frighten Rebecca or her classmates. These observations strengthened her resolve to hold steady in her expectations for Rebecca's school attendance. Yet, whenever she thought of being firm with Rebecca, she found herself in an almost unbearable state of anxiety, consumed with the sense that Rebecca really had good reason for fearing school. By the time she consulted a therapist, Ms. D felt immobilized; she could neither kindly but firmly send her daughter to school, nor comfortably allow her to stay at home.

In the initial session, Rebecca's mother spontaneously described a very upsetting event from her own elementary school days. She indicated that while she had never forgotten this incident, it did not usually occupy her thoughts. However, when the memory was triggered, it evoked shockingly powerful feelings. During her early elementary school years, one of her teachers had hit her for a minor infraction of the rules. She had suffered not only physical pain, but intense humiliation and fright. Because she was so worried that her parents would be furious with her for having gotten into trouble at school, she had not told them about this incident. Instead she feared that they might find out about it and punish her further, both for the misbehavior and for hiding it from them.

Although Rebecca had absorbed some of her mother's anxieties, it seemed as if she and her mother had been able to negotiate the preschool and kindergarten years, in part because her mother was allowed to spend significant amounts of time in the classroom. Her actual presence in the school offered Rebecca's mother a sense of safety. When she had to allow Rebecca more physical and emotional distance, her separation anxiety became almost unbearable.

Because she had not internalized an image of a protective, watchful parent, she could not instill that image of herself in her daughter. Rebecca came to share her mother's unconscious conviction that Rebecca could neither feel, nor actually be, safe except under her mother's actual, watchful eye. Ms. D intended her continued physical presence not only as a conscious and concrete reassurance to Rebecca but also as an unconscious reassurance to herself that she, unlike her own parents, was a concerned and protective mother.

Separation from her daughter triggered a state of psychological confusion in Ms. D. When Rebecca voiced the fears she had absorbed from her mother, Ms. D felt caught between contradictory identifications. She identified with Rebecca, who represented her own frightened childhood self. Consequently, she also identified with the view of herself she expected from Rebecca—a parent as distant, emotionally unavailable, and punitive as she had felt her own parents to be.

Since she had no stable, positive, internal representations of parents who could comfort a child, even from a distance, she could not bear the thought of separating herself from Rebecca. Her only choice was to identify with the sense of fear and helplessness she had unconsciously endowed in Rebecca. Then, if she could stay close, she could demonstrate that, contrary to her unconscious belief about herself, she was kind, caring, and available and distinctly different from her own parents.

Rebecca's approach to psychotherapy mirrored her approach to school—she would agree to go as long as her mother joined her. Because Ms. D could not resist Rebecca's anxious insistence that her mother accompany her down the short hallway to the office, Ms. D joined Rebecca in the first therapy session. About halfway through the session, at the therapist's suggestion, Ms. D returned to the waiting room. At that point, Rebecca's preoccupation with her mother's whereabouts began to interfere substantially with her spontaneous or pleasurable play.

For a number of reasons, Rebecca's therapist forcefully recommended that she return to school as soon as possible. He was convinced that the shared perception of danger was internally generated and that tolerating Rebecca's avoidance of school would serve only to reinforce its power as a phobic object. He was concerned that Rebecca's absences would begin to interfere with her finding a place for herself with the other children. He also feared that her mother's ongoing presence placed too strong a regressive pull not only on Rebecca, but also on the other children, which might lead them to shun Rebecca and her "babyishness" as a means of defending against their own longings for the mothers they had left behind.

To that end, following the second session with Rebecca, he met with her parents to plan her return to school. He suggested that he would meet with Rebecca the following day and, in that session, would continue to talk with her about her concerns about school while emphasizing that her parents and teachers agreed that the time had come for her to become a real first-grader, which meant leaving Mommy at home. He stressed the importance of her parents conveying their conviction that school was both a safe and enjoyable activity for Rebecca.

The parents and Rebecca's therapist agreed on a plan for reintro-
ducing Rebecca to school. On the morning following her third therapy
session, her father would accompany Rebecca to school. Ms. D and
the therapist would meet midmorning; Rebecca's teacher had agreed
to phone the mother over her lunch break. Following school that
afternoon, her mother would bring Rebecca in for therapy.

When her therapist saw Rebecca the following day, he continued
to articulate his clear grasp of and genuine appreciation for Rebecca's
struggle to enjoy herself either in the therapy office or at school when
she was so worried about her mother. Rebecca repeated her previous
reply: It wasn't that she didn't like school, she just liked it better with
her mother there. Her therapist suggested that it was often nice to
have one's mother along, but children just have to do some things on
their own, including going to school. He also noted that school
provides a very good place to do some of the things children like much
better than grown-ups. When he asked how Rebecca's mother liked
jumping rope, it brought the first smile he had seen to Rebecca's face.

The next day her father accompanied Rebecca to school. As they
approached the entrance, Rebecca asked her father if he would remain
with her if it was "too scary" to stay alone. He reminded her that
school was a safe and interesting place for children. He said he would
take her to her classroom and then go to his office. She tried again;
would he stay until noon? "No." How about until the first recess? "No,"
again. Would he stay for 5 minutes? "Yes."

Rebecca beamed. Five minutes into the morning, a little tearfully,
she hugged him good-bye.

While Rebecca was at school, Ms. D came for the scheduled
consultation. During the session she seemed anxiously embarrassed by
her concerns, principally that Rebecca would feel abandoned. The
therapist consistently reminded her that the little girl at school was
Rebecca, who had quite different parents from her own. Ms. D talked
about how grim and mean her teacher had been and how different
Rebecca's teachers were. The therapist noted this comparison and
gently wondered if she might be a little jealous at the idea that
Rebecca might enjoy school much more fully than she had. The idea
that she might want to join in Rebecca's fun intrigued Ms. D who had
previously felt only that going to school with Rebecca was far preferable to remaining at home, worrying about her daughter's suffering at
school.

The therapist suggested that when she couldn't see herself reflected in Rebecca's eyes, she worried that she resembled her own mother; she had trouble remembering, in her daughter's absence, that Rebecca held an image of her as an available, caring mother, not the harsh and punitive image of mother that Ms. D carried inside of her.

That afternoon when Ms. D brought Rebecca to her appointment, Rebecca calmly slid off her chair when her therapist entered the waiting room. With a shy smile she informed her mother that she would walk to the office by herself.

Rebecca and her mother show the unconscious power of an inadequately integrated abusive incident. The therapist's work with them illustrates the effective use of collateral work with parents on behalf of the child. Because Ms. D was not his patient, the therapist limited his interpretations to those he felt would enable Rebecca's mother to function more effectively as a parent. As Rebecca's therapist, he was primarily interested in mobilizing all of the resources available to his young patient. Her mother's emotional support, essential to this process, remained inaccessible until he had helped her clarify the impact of her own childhood experiences on her identification with both parent and child. The limited interpretations the therapist offered Rebecca's mother were not intended as substitutes for her own psychological explorations. He offered them to help her crystallize the internalized images of parent and child that were interfering with her effective parenting.

When a parent, for whatever reason, cannot hold to a sense of self-as-parent, truly collaborative work cannot occur. Such was the case with Max's parents who were increasingly unable to differentiate their son's injuries and pain from their own. His mother's despair over not having protected Max ballooned, gradually but steadily, into a sense of herself as the defective parent of an irreparably damaged child. The boundary between them, tenuous even prior to the abuse, steadily dissolved over the months following Billy's assault. Given her reaction to the mere thought of Max's pain, she could not respond to Max's need for an effective, competent parent. Instead, she attempted to comfort both of them by increasingly close contact, which unfortunately intensified Max's regressive defenses in the face of these overwhelming and confusing events. Max's somatic complaints grew in number and intensity; headaches and stomachaches became a routine part of his life and his relationship to his mother. Her ministrations to her sickly son increasingly isolated them from the rest of the family.

Max missed school so frequently that he risked failing; when he was ill, his mother would often arrange to take time off from work to stay with him. However, when Max asked his mother to drive on a field trip or help with a special school project during working hours, his mother would sadly decline, citing the amount of work she had missed because of Max's ill health.

Billy's molestation of Max produced different but equally powerful effects on Max's father, who experienced Billy's behavior as a personal assault—a narcissistic injury that defied understanding. His sense of betrayal left him massively hurt and in danger of a profound depression, which he warded off by assuring himself with unrelenting devotion that Billy had been adequately punished. Max had always longed for more attention from his father and had felt jealous of his father's interest in Billy; ironically, his father's response to the molestation merely underscored Max's conviction that his father cared more about Billy than about him.

Max's father continued to deal haphazardly with his children. A great believer in the value of physical activity and sports, he made sure to involve each of his children in a sport and spent considerable time searching for good coaches. He relied on his wife's secretary for a weekly schedule of their sports activities and attended as many as his business commitments would allow. However, his children were often late to games and practices and occasionally had been driven home by a coach because their father either forgot to pick them up or could not extricate himself from a business meeting.

Sadly, Max's parents were entirely unable to accept the help of his therapist or to consider the therapist's suggestion that they seek individual treatment. Work, and the demands their children's schedules made on their time, rendered them simply "too busy." Billy's behavior had left them exhausted and had increased the number and intensity of their responsibilities. Despite their assurances that they entirely supported Max's continuing in psychotherapy, they simply could not get him to appointments on a reliable basis. Like school and sports, Max's therapy just quietly unraveled. Over the next several years, his parents made regular calls to Max's therapist, wondering if Max should resume therapy. There were also periodic calls from other therapists who wanted information about Max's history. With each encounter, Max was described as increasingly constricted in both behavior and affective expression. His mother's tearful preoccupation and his father's concern with Billy's whereabouts continued relatively unabated.

Sometimes it is not the confusion or disintegration of internalized images that impedes parents' effective interventions with their child, but their own reticence to look inward—to consider that physical abuse or sexual molestation is fundamentally an internal experience, the effects of which can be ameliorated only through internal, that is, psychological processes. When parents' own needs to externalize cogwheel with their child's wish for external solutions to internal problems, the path toward understanding becomes both circuitous and arduous.

Joslyn

Joslyn spent her early years of elementary school in an all-girls' school. The years passed relatively uneventfully, although Joslyn sometimes complained of feeling left out of the groups of popular girls. During her eighth-grade year, the female physical education teacher was rumored to be "too friendly" with her students. Students complained that the teacher's congratulatory hugs were too frequent and too long. In general, she made them uncomfortable. Although Joslyn never directly complained that this teacher had made sexual advances or comments to her, she frequently said that she was uncomfortable around this particular woman, as well as some of the girls in her class, whom she thought were probably lesbian. At Joslyn's request, her parents decided to move her to a coed high school, rather than let her move with her class into the girls' high school.

The investigations of the charges against the teacher received a great deal of attention in the local media. Joslyn and her parents followed the news coverage closely. Although they openly criticized the school's handling of the circumstances, they consistently refused to be interviewed or to join in other parents' public statements. For several weeks, the school situation frequently emerged as a dinner-table topic, not only within the family, but with friends and acquaintances.

Joslyn finished the school year and enjoyed the family vacation and her usual stay at overnight camp. Though anxious about being the "new kid," she was eager to try a different school. After a few weeks at this institution, Joslyn complained to her parents that the kids at school were calling her a "dyke" and studiously avoiding her.

The principal confirmed that he had heard about a couple of these taunts and had dealt with them firmly. His impression was that most of the children had either openly welcomed Joslyn or tried to befriend her but that Joslyn had remained somewhat aloof from her new classmates. When Joslyn's mother sought therapy for her daughter, she told the therapist that she "knew" this would happen. She explained her conviction that because of all of the media attention, the other children would think that Joslyn had left her previous school because the physical education teacher had molested her. She *knew* they would assume that the teacher would not have been interested in Joslyn unless Joslyn were lesbian.

Clearly, there are many complex factors at work here, but I wish to indicate the prominent role of externalization in the attempts to manage confusing and conflicting sexual feelings. Of course the teacher may well have behaved inappropriately—the investigation was inconclusive—but this vignette illustrates a quiet collusion among a number of players aimed at avoiding a conscious awareness that the troubling sexual conflicts stem from internal, rather than external, sources.

Despite the lack of legal truth in this case, the psychological truth was that Joslyn did not experience herself to be in a sexually safe environment. Her parents' moving her to a new school implicitly supported her unspoken view that her discomfort stemmed from being in the company of homosexual women and girls. Her parents quite deliberately moved her into an environment offering her more opportunities for heterosexual contact as she moved toward adolescence.

However, in externalization, the threatening environment that one wants to leave behind magically replicates itself in new locations. Thus Joslyn found herself still concerned about homosexuality in her new school, but with one important difference. Having been identified as lesbian, or at least coming from a school associated in the media with homosexual activities, Joslyn provided a convenient repository for the uncomfortable sexual conflicts and longings of her new classmates. If they could assign their own homosexual, "weird," or confused feelings to Joslyn, then by avoiding her, they could hope to avoid the feelings she represented.

When the taunts continued and Joslyn's parents again approached the school, they felt that the principal was less sympathetic. He indicated that Joslyn was "bringing this on herself" by distancing herself from other students. We can partly credit the principal's view: Joslyn's behavior did make her seem different or "weird." Her own feelings of being unacceptable and not fitting in could now, in her mind, be explained by the other students' disliking her. This defensive stance allowed her to avoid confronting her own ambivalence over being part of or distant from the group.

Joslyn did, because of her own anxieties about her budding sexuality, allow herself to be victimized by her fellow students. The principal could then accurately say that she contributed to the hostilities directed toward her. However, in holding Joslyn primarily responsible for the problem, the principal failed to address the anxieties that fueled the other students' animosities.

Joslyn's wish to avoid a situation that makes her uncomfortable is understandable, as is her parents' wish to keep her in a physically and emotionally safe setting. However, if the sensed danger emanates solely from internal conflict, changing the environment rarely brings relief. Particularly if the issues that are driving the externalization, in this case conflicts over developing sexualities, touch a universal chord of unease, then the new environment may well replicate the old. We must recognize that a child who feels plagued by discomfitting impulses and affects may externalize these unacceptable conflicts onto the people around her and will consequently find herself in situations that are uncomfortably familiar. This does not mean that when we discover children in a physically, sexually, or emotionally abusive environment we do not make clear, unambiguous, and effective steps to change that environment, even if the child has in some way provoked her mistreatment.

In psychotherapeutic work with children, one must always be alert to the dangers of the parents' idealization of the therapist. This is particularly true in work with the parents of an abused child. Because both child and parents may have such an enormous investment in defensive externalization of the abuse, they tend toward a concomitant externalization of the solution to the problem. The unwary therapist can easily be seduced into the seemingly sensible but actually inappropriate role of consultant to a parent whose sense of efficacy has been shattered by the intrusion of an external danger into the parent–child relationship.

Mrs. R

Mrs. R contacted a child therapist regarding the baby-sitter who had been caring for her children, Stevie, a little over 3, and Natalie, about to celebrate her first birthday. She had just learned that Lisa, who had cared for her children for approximately 6 months had, with some regularity, spanked or threatened to spank them or smack their fingers.

Lisa had been dismissed promptly and Mrs. R was now preparing to interview new candidates to care for her young children. She explained that she wanted consultation in an effort to avoid her previous mistakes and to figure out how to protect her children from a recurrence of physical punishment. She had very specific questions that she hoped to address with the consultant, chiefly concerning how to devise interview strategies that would help identify sitters who relied on corporal punishment. Mrs. R also wanted to know how and when the children could safely be left with a sitter again.

On the face of it, Mrs. R's questions made perfectly sensible use of the therapist's expertise. However, had the therapist merely acquiesced in these requests for assistance, he would have unwittingly colluded with and promoted Mrs. R's sense of failure and inability to protect her children. When she sought consultation, Mrs. R had begun to internalize a sense of herself as an inadequate parent with profoundly impaired judgment. If the therapist had allowed this to stand unquestioned and unexplored, it might have produced far-reaching negative consequences on the parent–child relationship, as well as on both child and parent individually.

Rather than immediately offer the advice Mrs. R requested, the therapist asked to know a little about her children, other experiences they had had with sitters, how she had discovered the spankings, and what she and her husband had done when they learned about these punishments. Despite her tearful self-reproaches and self-doubts, it became increasingly clear as she talked that Mrs. R was an exceedingly bright and articulate woman, quite capable of devising "interview strategies" that would inform her about potential caretakers' attitudes toward discipline. When the consultant offered this observation, Mrs. R went on to explain that because Lisa, the sitter, had seemed depressed and rather brittle, she and her husband had already made a decision to replace her.

It was in the context of exploring Stevie's reaction to the possibility of a new sitter that their young son had said he wanted someone who didn't hit him. This confirmed their sense that something had been amiss in Lisa's care of their children and mortified them. When his parents asked Stevie if he wanted to say good-bye to Lisa, he said they "could just write her a letter." That evening they had phoned Lisa to tell her that they would no longer be needing her services; they had also phoned Child Protective Services, not because they felt that Lisa's behavior actually reached the level of reportable child abuse, but because they wanted to know whether a registry for nannies or professional sitters existed, so that other parents might be alerted to her behavior.

As the consultant heard more about the ways in which these parents had responded to their children, particularly the older child, he was impressed with the disparity between the actuality of the mother's emotional attunement to and effectiveness with her children and her self-perceptions. He verbalized a simple, straightforward observation that the sitter's behavior seemed to have seriously undermined Mrs. R's sense of herself as a good parent. As she went on to talk about her concern that this incident would have a lasting effect on her son's capacity to trust others, Mrs. R also recognized that this worry had to do with her feeling that her son couldn't trust his parents to care for him.

This example illustrates the enormous impact even an apparently relatively minor violation of a child's well-being can have on a parent. In this case, the parents appeared to be more strongly affected than the child.

They acted swiftly to remove their children from a noxious environment. Because they were able to absorb Stevie's concerns and translate them into effective action, his environment was quickly transformed into one in which he felt safe. Even though they were quite distressed, his parents' actions on his behalf were not exaggerated by their own anxieties; the internalized images they carried of themselves as competent parents were shaken but not destroyed. Because the consultant recognized this, he was able to help them reestablish a more functional view of themselves relatively quickly rather than collude with an emerging view of themselves as inadequate, inattentive, or incompetent.

I have confined the above discussion to therapeutic work with parents whose child has been or was thought to have been abused by someone outside the family. In these cases, one must assess the possibility of establishing a primarily collaborative relationship with the parents on behalf of the child's emotional well-being. Of course, like Amy's and Rebecca's mothers, parents often do and should derive therapeutic benefit from working with the child's therapist, even though that is not the primary purpose of the relationship.

However, depending on the abusive circumstances, children may be brought to treatment by one or both parents, a relative who is serving as either a temporary or permanent guardian, or a nonrelative foster parent or guardian. Those cases in which one or both parents have been identified as perpetrators, yet retain custody of the abused child(ren), can prove extremely complex, not only because of the individual and family dynamics. Because of their emotional problems and the probability of their ongoing involvement with one or more social service agencies or legal processes it may be difficult or impossible to establish truly collaborative relationships with these parents. Collaboration suggests cooperation among relative equals; parents whose access to their children is determined by the courts are, themselves, indirectly dependents of the court. They can cooperate with the child's therapist, but they cannot act in true and independent partnership.

With substitute parents, whether adoptive, related, or unrelated foster parents, the child encounters more players in both his internal and external world. Along with the substitutes, his original parents occupy a very important place in his affective life, even when they no longer act in his day-to-day world. However, beyond mere quantity, the significance of the absent parent in the circumstances of the abuse often raises highly loaded issues with multiple and complex implications for therapists and substitute parents. If the reason for a biological parent's separation from the child stems from either the infliction of abuse or the failure to protect the child, the temptation to vilify the absent parent can be most seductive.

If, for a variety of unconscious reasons, the abused child steadfastly draws the substitute caregiver into an abusive relationship, the absent perpetrator can easily be blamed for the child's behavior, as well as for the substitute parent's response. For example, Damien who was placed in foster care as a consequence of his parents' abuse and neglect, consistently cowered in response to his foster mother's ministrations and directives. Initially she correctly understood his response to her as an indication of how his parents had treated him. Because she genuinely cared about this little boy and never hit or screamed at him, it took longer for her to see the ways in which her rather abrasive manner contributed to Damien's reactions to her.

The compelling explanatory power of abuse in a child's background can pose real roadblocks to careful examination of the more subtle contributions that caregiver and child make to their ongoing relationship. For instance, a foster mother explains a child's physical attacks on other children as resulting from the beatings he received from his father. She fails to consider that, in the face of his misbehavior, her repeated threats to send him to a different home might contribute to his anxiety and acting out. In another case, the sister who is raising her drug-addicted brother's children continually reassures them that their father will get better and that they'll return to him. She speaks from her own guilt-driven misperceptions of the severity of his problems, not recognizing that their depression stems more from feeling rejected by her than from a wish to be reunited with their father. Clearly, there are countless permutations of the relationships that make up the world of the abused child who has been removed from the care of his biological parents.

The ways in which parents or the adults responsible for an abused child approach psychotherapy frequently differ subtly from the attitudes of parents who come for other reasons. Although parents typically have numerous motivations and silent agendas, the parents or guardians of an abused child often convey that they want the therapist to somehow undo the abuse, to find it and ferret it out—just simply to remove it from the child's life.

Therapists who treat children recognize that when parents request an evaluation of their child's symptoms, they almost always have a wish, sometimes verbalized, that the child will be found healthy and not in need of treatment. If we remind them that not every symptomatic child requires psychotherapy, it often visibly relieves them. However, this frequently is not the case for parents of children who have been sexually molested or physically abused. Hearing that not all children who have experienced sexual or physical assault require treatment seems to intensify, rather than diminish, their anxiety. How do we understand this? In particular, how do we understand it alongside the parallel, although apparently contradictory, phenomenon of parents who refuse to acknowledge the horrible impact of an assaultive experience on their child, even when the child is obviously suffering and grossly symptomatic?

I believe this seeming paradox, along with many other aspects of child abuse and treatment, can be understood by recognizing the enormous ambivalence over recognizing the fact of abuse as an *internal* experience. Parents, both on their own behalf and in collusion with their child, feel a powerful wish to maintain the abuse as an external event, which can somehow be eradicated, forgotten, or undone or explained away. Some parents contend that any abuse their child suffered doesn't mean much at all; other parents want the therapist to eradicate any meaning abuse might have for their child. Thus, the parents who refuse to bring their children for psychological evaluation perhaps do not differ greatly in their stance from the parents who see psychotherapy as an inevitable consequence of abuse.

The parents who cannot hear that their child may not need treatment sometimes seem to expect that the therapist will reverse or remove the effects of the abuse. They have trouble imagining that the child's internal organization and identifications may not have been irreparably damaged by the abuse, or that the child, with their help, can muster the emotional resources to manage the internal reorganization and identification demanded by the abusive experience. Instead, the parent sees the experience as an external event that must be cured by an external source, in this case the therapist. This position in some ways parallels that of the parents who insist that, since the abuse was something that happened *to* a child, once it has stopped, it will have no consequences on the child's inner life and therefore does not require the intervention of a psychological expert.

From the above, it should be obvious that when parents or caregivers consider psychotherapy on behalf of an abused child, they bring with them many spoken and unspoken expectations. They may both simultaneously—consciously and unconsciously—view themselves and the therapist in multiple, changeable, and contradictory roles. The conscious, often overlapping roles that important adults play can be difficult for the child and therapist to grasp; the unconscious place each holds in the world of the child's internal objects requires time for quiet reflection to be fully appreciated and understood. Because the varying roles the child assigns to the substitute parent(s) and therapist may very well change over time, the players can easily be drawn to enacting the parts assigned them in the child's internal drama. The therapist must be watchful, lest the adults allow themselves to be pitted against each other in the child's attempt to reconcile himself to a growing awareness that the world is not easily divided into "good guys" and "bad guys."

Chapter *T*en

The Unconscious
Transmission of Abuse

Although almost unfathomable, in our work we inevitably encounter parents who seem to need to have an abused child. Often, although not always, they were themselves victims of child abuse, but neither in childhood nor adulthood have they received successful treatment. Sometimes they seem unwittingly, but repeatedly, to put their children in the path of danger. In other instances they become so preoccupied with protecting the child from the dangers outside the family that they cannot even consider any negative influence they might have on their child. Other parents unconsciously use the child to contain feelings they find intolerable; paradoxically, in their efforts to protect the child, they come to fear the child. Particularly, a parent who him- or herself has been abused may find it exceedingly difficult, despite his very best intentions, to avoid abusive behavior. This stems not simply from learned social and neurological patterns but from a profound jealousy of his or her child who has a chance to enjoy the good parent who existed only in his or her own childhood dreams.

Gary

Gary's father had routinely whipped him with his leather belt. Minor disobedience earned a couple of lashes on his clothed buttocks or legs, while major infractions were met with lashings on bare skin that often left welts and sometimes drew blood. Gary was determined not to repeat this abusive behavior with his child, but he increasingly found himself enraged by the obstinacy of his young son. With sadness and confusion, he described the way he disciplined this very active little boy.

First, he would issue a warning about any misbehavior. If that didn't work, Bobby would be given a time-out on a chair. If he resisted, he would be sent to his room. Any further protests were met with Gary's removing his belt and threatening to hit Bobby. Gary reported that he had given a great deal of thought to this plan and, for quite a while had been pleased that he had never "had" to strike Bobby, but recently, Bobby had responded to this threat by hitting his father. Feeling defeated and completely at his wits' end, Gary gave Bobby a demonstration of a whipping, by mildly swatting the little boy's legs. Bobby became even more frantic. The terror in his son's eyes made his father call for help.

Gary understood and recoiled from the pain of the physical punishments he had endured as a child. It was harder for him to grasp the anguish he suffered from the ever present threats of beatings. Because his only model for discipline involved a ruthless abuse of power, he really didn't know how to assert his parental authority without resorting to aggression. Unwittingly, his threats to hit Bobby terrified and provoked his young son; his attempts to limit Bobby's misbehavior only caused it to escalate.

With his therapist's help, Gary was able to recognize the frightening power of his threats, even if he rarely acted on them. He also came to appreciate how much he envied Bobby his good father and how upsetting he found Bobby's seeming lack of appreciation for his efforts. With sadness and anger, he wondered why his own father couldn't see the terror and pain in his eyes. From this vantage point, rather than threatening his son with the belt, Gary began to reassure Bobby that there would be no more hitting. Gary had to withstand several weeks of rather dramatic testing of limits before Bobby seemed able to accept his father's statements that he simply would not hit Bobby—that they could always find another way of helping him to learn how to control himself.

When Gary could recognize the abusive nature of his behavior and the complexity of its relationship to his own childhood experiences, he could begin to look for other strategies for helping his son.

Previously, he had simply refrained from hitting, with little confidence that his parental authority stemmed from Bobby's love for rather than fear of him.

In some instances, the child may fall victim to abuse from someone outside the family, despite a parent's careful attention. Once the child has become an identified victim, the parent may be unable to see the child as anything other than a victim of abuse. Particularly if she herself was abused as a child and her essential identity remains structured around the abuse, her children, through identification risk also seeing themselves as victims. These cases pose particular therapeutic problems because these parents typically have the greatest investment in maintaining and perpetuating the externalization of the abusive experience, the most strenuous resistance to recognizing their contributions to the child's ongoing difficulties, and the greatest narcissistic vulnerability to feeling accused of being abusive. Because abuse requires both victim and perpetrator, child and parent can easily become enmeshed in reciprocal enactments in which they alternately identify with the victimized child or the abusive adult.

Magda and David

I was the fourth of a long line of clinicians Magda consulted about her son, David. With impressively flamboyant gestures, Magda described her adolescence in Eastern Europe during World War II. It seemed a story that she had told many times before and would probably tell many times again. Her family had barely escaped the Nazi invasion; they found refuge in France with "friends of friends" who gave them a place to stay until they could immigrate to the United States. During their several months in France, the man with whom they were staying regularly visited Magda in her bed. She endured intercourse with him because she "didn't know what else to do." She didn't tell her parents because they were depressed and preoccupied. She didn't know what would become of her family if they had to leave this home. She felt they had no other place to go, and this was the price she had to pay.

Many years later, when David was about 3, Magda left him with a trusted friend, John, who lived in their building. After a few hours she returned home to find David sobbing and her friend uncharacteristically eager to leave. Magda eventually concluded that John had masturbated against David's buttocks. When she picked him up she found that "his back was still wet from the ejaculation."

Magda went screaming though the halls to confront John but could find him nowhere in the building. However, by the time she returned to her apartment, all of the neighbors knew what had happened. Magda immediately took David for a physical exam and filed a report with Child Protective Services. David had short-term psychotherapy through this program, which Magda did not think very helpful, since David was seen by an intern. From there she went to a clinic, without much more satisfaction. Her main complaint seemed to be that David wouldn't talk about the sexual abuse, and the therapists didn't seem to find it necessary. Magda believed that talking was the only way he would recover, so she talked about it with him on a regular basis.

A few years later, when he was about 8, Magda again tried therapy because of David's lack of attentiveness in school and quiet isolation at home. After 2 years, she discontinued treatment with that therapist because "All they did was play. David wasn't getting any better."

When I spoke with this therapist, he described his futile efforts to get Magda into her own treatment. He agreed that not much had happened in his 2-year treatment of David, but he did feel that David looked forward to their sessions as a quiet refuge from his mother's relentless verbal assaults and efforts to get him to remember and talk about the sexual abuse he had suffered at the age of 3. David said he didn't remember anything about it, so he had nothing to talk about.

Magda did not waver in her conviction that David's problems stemmed from the incident with the babysitter. In trying to impress upon me the importance of David's seeing a therapist who would insist that David confront these issues, she described the following episode with bone-chilling serenity. While waiting for a bus, she had tried to strike up a conversation with her son. David's typically taciturn response infuriated her. She explained to him that this was exactly the reason he needed to see a therapist; until he could talk about being sexually assaulted, he'd never be able to talk about anything else important. David began to move away from her. She described how this forced her to chase him down the street, "talking louder and louder to make him listen" to her explanations about the source of his problems.

Magda's picture of a 10-year-old boy standing on a street corner while his mother loudly lamented the damage he suffered from having

John's "semen spread all over" left me horrified. Magda showed no sign of embarrassment nor any empathy for the humiliation that this public display might have caused David.

Magda's opinion was clear and unchanging: "It's what you can't talk about that hurts you." Magda was distressed when I told her that I would not see David unless she also began psychotherapy. She explained that she had already had an analysis many years ago which she had found "a complete waste of time" for rather vague reasons. She seemed to feel that she had successfully manipulated the analyst into allowing her to talk about "whatever nonsense" came into her head. However, she accepted the name of the therapist I suggested. A few months later, she called to tell me the referral I had made was no good, and she was looking on her own.

Magda continues to call me periodically to see if I have time available or for the name of a therapist for herself or David. At one point, her description of David's behavior suggested that he should be seen for an immediate evaluation, which I did not have time to do. I gave her the names of three outstanding therapists. She called back to tell me that two of them had no time and the other must not be very good because he had openings.

Magda always insists that the therapists call me and always gives me her opinion of the people I have referred her to. Sometimes she is so offended by a comment or a phone call not returned quickly enough that she calls to let me know this person just may not be as good as I think. Or she may allow David several months of therapy before breaking off the treatment for predictable reasons.

Over the years, I have struggled to understand Magda's attachment to me in a way that would allow me to be helpful to her. She had been given my name by the director of the first clinic where David had been treated and became quite fond of this woman, who had done the initial assessment of mother and child, even though she expressed disapproval of the therapist there. Over the course of David's treatment at the clinic, Magda would sometimes "drop in for a chat" with the director. She valued these conversations for their intimacy and her sense that the director appreciated her opinion. They seemed to offer an antidote to the humiliation she suffered by having her son seen by an intern at a clinic.

Because of the source of the referral, Magda came to me with an idealized transference; because, like the director of the clinic, I was not entirely available, I became a more valued object. I believe that her wish to preserve me as a reliable, though unavailable, object explained why she never asked to have her own therapy with me. Keeping me at a distance protected both of us from the disappointments that sustained contact in any relationship inevitably brought.

Over the years that Magda has maintained this distant contact, I have worried about the impact on David of starting and stopping relationships with so many different therapists and wondered whether I should simply refuse to collude with Magda's unconscious need to destroy any real chance for David to get help. When Magda once told me that she had gotten so fed up with "shrinks" that she had taken David to a psychic healer, I recognized the sense of helplessness that underlay my omnipotent fantasy that I could change her behavior by simply refusing to participate in it.

At least Magda keeps in touch and allows me to give some shape to her impossible search to find help for herself and her child. From our phone contacts, our occasional meetings, and Magda's insistence that I speak with every therapist to whom I have referred her, I have accumulated a great deal of information about Magda. Although I can only speculate, I believe her search is futile for a number of reasons. First, Magda experiences herself and David as having been dirtied by the sexual abuse they suffered; she does not expect that anyone can tolerate being close to either of them. Before a therapist can become as disgusted by David as she is with herself, she becomes disgruntled and leaves. Believing them both to be truly beyond help, she must repeatedly demonstrate the inefficacy of therapy, lest she develop hope and risk having it shattered. I have also come to wonder whether she is genuinely afraid of losing David to mental health. Only if he is defective would he want to be with her, and she cannot bear to lose him. Her ambivalence about saving her child does propel her repeatedly to seek help for him, but that same ambivalence renders her unable to tolerate the possibility of his developing meaningful relationships. The repeated losses of relationships would certainly contribute to David's keeping an emotional distance from each new therapist, but his sense that his attachment to his mother depends on his being a defective victim may be an even more powerful factor.

Magda tolerates my curiosity about why it is so difficult for her to find help for herself or David; she quickly dismisses any psychological explanations I might offer, but in a few weeks or months she calls for more. Perhaps she simply cannot get any closer right now. I hope that these tiny morsels may eventually allow her to satisfy her hunger for self-knowledge. As for David, I simply have to trust that these relatively benign, if not terribly useful, therapeutic encounters will keep open the possibility of psychotherapy when he reaches adulthood. At the very least, he will have spent a significant amount of time sitting with people who do not find him disgusting, can tolerate his need for emotional distance, can be thoughtful about his feelings and the motivations for his behavior, and do not feel compelled to intrude into areas that he has not invited them to examine. But maybe this represents wishful thinking on my part; these fragments of pseudo-therapy may be accomplishing nothing at all.

That David actually had been abused allowed Magda to organize her own self-loathing around the damage she perceived in both herself and her son. Although she could sometimes fleetingly acknowledge the inappropriateness of her behavior toward David, Magda could quickly retreat to John's actual attack as an explanation for David's difficulties. Once she had moved into this position, she grew impervious to any exploration of her possible contribution to her child's problems. Magda's real terror that her own defectiveness would inevitably damage her child forced her to look elsewhere for an explanation for his difficulties, lest she discover the real "truth"—that she herself was totally responsible for his suffering. Sadly and ironically, of course, this external focus made ameliorating the conflicts in the ongoing parent–child relationship impossible.

Magda exemplifies the parent who relies on a history of actual physical or sexual abuse to shield her from her unconscious fears of harming her child. Other parents may unconsciously use their child to protect them from powerful unconscious fears of damaging aggression; that is, in order to avoid becoming an abusive parent, the parent unconsciously creates an abusive child.

When these families first seek consultation, they often present the main issue simply as their difficulty in setting appropriate limits. Children are described as out of control and disobedient. Upon closer examination, it becomes evident that there are no clear rules—or else, every rule has so many exceptions that neither parent nor child can keep them straight. In such cases, basic education about children's developmental needs and capabilities sometimes enables parents to set and maintain appropriate expectations. Happily, when the parents can be helped to understand that aggression, per se, is not dangerous but an integral aspect of human behavior, they can recognize the benefits of setting and firmly holding to reasonable limits. Their realization that this expression of aggression does not harm their child, but forms a necessary part of successful parenting sometimes allows for family tensions to be resolved relatively easily and without psychotherapy.

In cases where parent–child interactions are more tinged with psychopathology, a psychoeducational approach rarely works. Instead of enjoying the successes that a therapist's suggestions might offer, some parents must unconsciously undermine any and every bit of advice that does not confirm their view of themselves as inadequate parents or their children as damaged, defective, or ungrateful off-spring.

When a parent's terror of her own aggression is so overwhelming that she cannot tolerate its entering into consciousness, parent and child can easily become ensnared in a web of physical and verbal abuse. In these families, overly permissive parenting provides the only mechanism the parent can devise to protect the child from her own lethally aggressive impulses. Unfortunately, when allowed to remain unconscious, the impulses will inevitably be acted upon by either parent or child—and sometimes by both.

Nina and Colin

Nina presented Colin for evaluation and treatment shortly after his fifth birthday. She expressed concern that he was depressed and distressed following the separation and impending divorce of Nina and her husband, Greg. Although he did not accompany her to the initial appointment, she assured me that Colin's father would cooperate with the evaluation and be "relatively supportive" of any therapy.

Nina had been in therapy for most of her 30-some years. As a child, she had been rebellious, which she now understood as a means of trying to manage considerable anxiety in the face of an exacting and overly critical father and overly indulgent mother. Nina tried to imitate her father's shrewd, ambitious attitudes, but these traits didn't come easily to her. Her attempts to identify with him tended to show themselves in her arbitrary, but excessive demands for control. Because she felt she could not measure up to her father's expectations, Nina preferred to think of herself as "free-spirited," like her mother. Both her mother's and Nina's "flightiness" enraged her father. He saw the break-up of her marriage as one more predictable example of her poor judgment, inability to stick with anything, and impossibly inane approach to life.

As Nina described her present and past life, her pervasive sense of emptiness became increasingly apparent. She still seemed to be bouncing between unintegrated internal images of her father and mother. She described giving dinner parties that she had planned to the tiniest detail; afterwards she would collapse in anxiety and exhaustion. Her children were dressed to perfection and attended the right classes, schools, and parties. They had only to express a mild interest in a toy for it to appear. She laughed that she knew that she wasn't supposed to "spoil" them but found it very hard to resist, especially since the separation had been so hard on them.

Not surprisingly, beneath the veneer of perfection, things were a frightful mess. The exquisitely decorated house was always strewn with children's clothes, toys, candy wrappers, and uneaten food. Long after the children and housekeeper had gone to bed, Nina would be up cleaning and trying to restore order. She told the children they had to pick up their toys, but they didn't listen. She explained that they had to sit at the table for meals, but they just got up and took their food with them. She briefly tried withholding dessert until they finished dinner. They helped themselves.

Initially Nina adopted a rather blasé attitude toward this. She reported these examples with a kind of "kids will be kids" tolerance. Interestingly, she showed extremely good judgment in her selection of books on parenting and child development. Nina was a bright, well-educated woman who knew that these readings provided little help to her, but she could not understand why. Although she tried to follow the suggestions of friends, teachers, pediatricians, and experts in child development, nothing seemed to work. Nina certainly had the cognitive capability to try new strategies in child raising, but her underlying rage toward her children demanded that she destroy any positive moves she or they made.

Greg, Colin's father, was an articulate, unassuming man, whom Nina quite consciously chose because of his apparent dissimilarity to her father. Initially he had been attracted to Nina's vibrancy and "take-charge" attitude. However, he came to see her vivaciousness as intolerable flightiness and her competence as a thin mask for a pathologically excessive attention to detail. By way of example, he explained that for all of his adult life he had had toast and coffee for breakfast. That's all he wanted. When they were first married, Nina insisted on preparing him a "real" breakfast and would get up an hour before he did to surprise him with homemade pancakes or muffins and fresh fruit. Sometimes these efforts were successful, but much of the time Nina was distraught because something had gone wrong. He would spend the time he had set aside for breakfast calming and comforting her, trying to reassure her that she had not ruined his day. He found his attempts just to have toast and coffee futile. Gradually he either scheduled or invented more and more early-morning meetings. By the time of the separation, he usually left the house before the rest of the family awoke.

Greg had grown up in a house much like the one Nina was trying to create. He loathed it and felt that a measure of the success of his therapy was his ability to tolerate some disorder without overwhelming anxiety. He took the children's lack of concern for orderliness and manners as a sign of healthy independence. As a child, he had been too worried about upsetting his parents to risk doing anything other than what they wanted. He explained that his parents had traveled a great deal; when they were at home, they often spent evenings out. Because he spent much of his childhood feeling "lost, alone, and sad," he was particularly sensitive to Colin's mood, which did seem depressed to him.

At the time the family contacted me, Colin was 5 years old, his sister, Nancy, was 7, and his younger brother, Drew, almost 2. Nancy had been in therapy for about 2 years, from about ages 4 to 6, because of numerous, almost incapacitating fears. Nina was considering contacting the therapist because Nancy was again having trouble falling asleep and complaining of bad dreams. Nina saw Drew as an exceptionally willful child; Greg thought he was a perfectly normal, exuberant toddler.

While Greg felt that he had been driven out of the family by Nina's excessive demands and bossiness, Nina felt that Greg had simply been too self-involved to meet the basic needs of the children. Their ongoing battles over food typified their inability to compromise or to respond empathically to the anxieties behind each other's position.

Nina insisted that the children eat healthily and with good manners. She allowed no prepared foods in the house and carefully rationed all sweets. The table was meticulously and properly set for all meals. Greg cringed at these requirements because of their association to his own unhappy childhood. He urged Nina to allow the children an occasional pizza or trip to a fast-food restaurant. Nina responded by organizing a pizza party for the children and their friends; she spent the day making whole wheat pizza crust and chopping vegetables so that they could have a selection of healthy toppings. Greg took this as a mockery of his attempts to offer the children a simple, uncomplicated meal.

Nina could not understand that Greg liked casual dinners at the kitchen table because they figured among the few pleasant memories he had of his childhood. Greg could not understand that Nina's insistence on formal, "healthy" dining represented her efforts to counteract the neglect and isolation she had felt as a child. Indeed, there was truth in the perceptions each had of the other. Each saw the other as unable to control the children, particularly Colin, although they had vastly different explanations for their behavior. When Greg took the children out for a meal, which he did frequently, he provided them with an endless supply of money for video games in order to ward off any irritability or tantrums. Nina felt this excessive indulgence reflected Greg's reluctance to set any limits on the children. He defended his behavior as a simple attempt to allow the children to relax and have a good time. When Nina read to the children at dinner, Greg saw this as her excessive need for control. She defended her behavior as providing an enriched environment for her children.

Nina initially described Colin extremely sympathetically. She saw him as a depressed child who was suffering the effects of an unpleasant parental divorce. She felt that Colin, in particular, responded strongly to the effects of his father's emotional and physical withdrawal from the family. Colin's kindergarten teacher also described him as sad and withdrawn. She worried that the increased demands for attention and performance would leave him lost in first grade.

Colin's behavior in the initial sessions reflected his mother's and teacher's descriptions. He was listless and showed little interest in the toys. Much of the time he seemed to move into a world of daydreams, staring out the window with a far-away look in his eyes. I commented that he acted like a boy with a lot on his mind. He shrugged. Over the course of the first several weeks, I talked with him about how his mommy and daddy were still fighting even though they lived in two different houses now. He generally offered some indication of assent but added little to my comments. During this time Colin happily greeted me at the beginning of each session. He began to offer some mild protest about having to leave, usually by finding a reason to extend an activity or prepare a toy for his return visit.

As therapy continued, Nina frequently called to let me know how much Colin loved coming to see me and how greatly his mood had improved as a result of his therapy. I agreed with her assessment that Colin's mood had brightened; he also played more freely and easily with me and at school. His teacher's worries about his getting lost in first grade were allayed. She now described Colin as a child who was "more tightly wound than other children." My attempts to address Nina's idealized transference, which would allow for no anger, disappointment, or distrust of me, had little effect. I was not much more successful in finding ways that she could allow herself more flexibility in her parenting.

Unfortunately, Nina's terror of not being a good mother made it almost impossible for her to lessen the demands she made on herself and her children. Her anxiety also substantially impaired her capacity to recognize that others did not always appreciate her efforts. For example, Nina proudly described inviting another mother with a child Drew's age over for the afternoon. She had planned the time to the most minute detail, including renting a popular video about toy trains, preparing lunch with a train motif, and developing an elaborate art activity around trains. She had scheduled a baby-sitter to take over the art activity so that the mothers could enjoy a luncheon, which had been equally carefully planned. Not unexpectedly, Nina's afternoon did not go as planned. The children had wandered off during the video, the other little boy had no interest in leaving his mother to spend time with a strange babysitter, and the other mother left early because her child was tired.

As Nina talked about the events that had led up to this most disappointing afternoon, I sensed that the other mother had tried in several ways to tell Nina that her plans were too elaborate for 2-year-olds and that she was also feeling a little overwhelmed with all of the preparations for what she had assumed was a simple afternoon of playing and chatting. Nina had also not been able to take in my gentle questions about the developmental appropriateness of her plans. Sadly, Nina masked the confusion and hurt of the afternoon behind anger at the rudeness and ingratitude of the other mother, who did not reciprocate. Indeed, it seemed that Colin and Drew were not invited to play at other children's homes as often as one would expect, given that their teachers described them as popular and sought after by other children.

The months of trying to function as a single parent began to take their toll on Nina and her relationship with her children. During this time, Nina had tried working with several well-respected clinicians, all of whom she found wanting. She sometimes thought Drew should begin therapy, as well.

An angry edge began to appear in Nina's voice, along with a desperation about getting any real help. When raising questions or requesting advice about discipline and limit-setting, Nina frequently prefaced her descriptions of difficulties at home with an announcement that she had talked to many professionals and friends and had already "tried everything and nothing works." Mealtimes continued to provide fertile ground for the ongoing battles. Nina complained that she could not keep the children at the table; reading to them had worked for a while, but now they all wanted a different book, and Drew insisted on sitting in her lap. Colin protested that if Drew didn't have to sit at the table, he wouldn't either. Nancy just picked up her plate and went to her room. Nina had tried enticing the children to meals by cooking each child's favorite foods. If they weren't hungry or otherwise didn't appreciate the incredible efforts she made to please them, Nina felt confused and hurt.

On the advice of a friend, one morning Nina announced that there would be no food other than at mealtimes and that all meals would be eaten at the table. Whether just bad luck or bad timing drawn from unconscious motives, that afternoon Colin went home with a classmate after school. Nina picked him up from this outing and on the way home enthusiastically described how she had spent the day making all of his favorite foods. Colin mumbled that he had stopped for pizza with his friend and really wasn't very hungry.

In this context, the facade of the perfect family finally shattered. Although it was impossible to reconstruct the events of that evening, Nina apparently decided to persevere with her plan for bringing order to the children's mealtimes. She arrived home in a rage and called the mother who had fed Colin pizza to complain about both her choice and timing of snacks, ending the conversation with the declaration that Colin would never play with her son again if this woman couldn't respect her rules.

Despite Colin's saying he wasn't hungry, Nina served dinner at the usual time, reminding him that, if he didn't eat, he couldn't have any food until breakfast. When Colin "just pushed his food around on his plate," Nina reached to remove it, and Colin knocked the plate to the floor. Colin ran to his room with Nina in pursuit. A physical struggle ensued, culminating in Colin's giving his mother a bloody nose.

In the aftermath, Colin said that he didn't mean to knock the food on the floor, he just pushed his mother's hand away because he was afraid she was going to hit him. Sometime in the course of this battle, in an effort to protect herself against Colin's kicks and slaps, Nina had pinned him to the floor and was sitting on him. Trying to struggle free, Colin hit his mother in the face, causing her nose to bleed quite profusely.

For the next few months Nina complained that Colin was "always" calling her names and hitting and kicking her, often without provocation. She described feeling entirely helpless and controlled by this child. The only thing that seemed to stop his attacks were her threats to leave. Colin would then calm down and cling to her, sometimes refusing to go to school out of a fear that his mother would not be at home when he returned. At school, Colin appeared depressed and distractible. In therapy, he returned to a state of listlessness, with little to say. He consistently said that he did not hit his mother, that "she made it up."

During this time, Nina would periodically drop the children at their father's house, with an announcement that he could try raising them for a while. She would typically reappear a few days later to fetch them home. On one occasion, Nina did not appear in the expected time frame. Greg called her house only to discover that the phone had been disconnected. A few days later a letter from Nina arrived saying that she could not tolerate the abuse and ingratitude of her children any longer, that they were now Greg's to raise.

Like any clinical vignette, this story omits much more about the individual and family dynamics than it includes. I use it to illustrate the creation of an abusive child. Nina's murderous impulses so terrified her that she could not tolerate bringing them into conscious awareness. Instead, she projected them onto those around her; eventually Colin became the prime repository for her hatefulness and self-loathing. Nina also found her profound feelings of inadequacy and imperfection intolerable. She attempted to keep them at bay by becoming the perfect mother whose children would reflect her idealized view of herself and them. Of course, like every child and parent, both Nina and her children were flawed: they made mistakes; they created disappointments; they fell short of expectations; and they became angry.

Unfortunately, Nina's internal world did not contain much room for modulated affects; there was little space between perfect and despicable. When she saw or imagined perfect love and adoration reflected in Colin's eyes, all was well. When there was any indication of a negative affect, she became terrified that Colin wanted to kill her—the imperfect parent. Indeed, Colin did become physically abusive toward his mother. While he denied it, others had witnessed his kicking, hitting, and spitting at her. He had little choice except to defend himself in an unconscious life-and-death struggle with his mother.

Although many professionals were involved in Nina's life, we had little more power than Colin to end this battle. Like children who cannot fully narrate their internal dramas (see Chapter 5), Nina had to rely on action to tell her story. Unfortunately, her children became unwitting actors in this tragedy, which could only end in the death or destruction of one of the players. Whether conscious or not, I believe Nina abandoned her children in order to save their lives and protect, as best she could, some shred of herself as an idealized parent. A bright, well-educated woman, Nina, of course, knew that her abandonment would be harmful to her children; however, she simply could not tolerate seeing her imperfection reflected in their eyes and behavior. Her absence freed her and them to imagine how wonderful things might have been if she had stayed.

Chapter *Eleven*

The Interface between Legal and Psychodynamic Considerations

The psychoanalytic treatment of any child must begin with an evaluation. Whether formally or informally, the clinician assesses the feasibility of undertaking intensive, perhaps lengthy psychotherapy with the child. Many, many factors go into the assessment. Foremost is the question of whether the child's essential difficulty is psychological. If so, the question remains as to whether psychotherapy will help to address the issues that brought the child to evaluation. Even if the child is experiencing intense psychological pain, that pain it may not be significantly reduced by psychotherapy until or unless other conditions are met. For example, it simply may not be possible for anyone to get the child to treatment. Thus, however complex the evaluation for treatment, essentially it must answer only two basic questions: namely, is psychoanalytic psychotherapy indicated, and can the environment support it?

Typically, the clinician is dealing only with the child and his or her immediate family in making this determination. However, when abuse has been alleged or demonstrated, the scope and meaning of an evaluation changes dramatically. A civil case may raise the question of monetary claims; whether determined by a jury or settled out of court, the issues may involve financial compensation for alleged or actual damages. In a criminal case, a child's credibility as a witness may be at issue. In either of these instances, mental health professionals may be called upon to evaluate the veracity of a child's statements. In a civil suit the evaluation may include an assessment of the extent of psychological damage, prognosis, and the likely course of the child's psychotherapy throughout childhood, adolescence, and adulthood. This information may be used to help the parties to arrive at mutually agreeable financial compensation.

A family or juvenile court most frequently orders an evaluation to help it address questions concerning the child's relationship to his or her immediate family, whether parents or substitute caretakers. At issue may be questions of the nature and quality of a child's attachments, legal or physical custody, the ability of the parent(s) to care for a child, and the child's developmental needs in relation to the emotional and physical capacities of the parent(s).

A court-ordered evaluation in response to allegations of physical or sexual abuse of a child will likely come at a time when the child has already been physically separated from the alleged perpetrator. The child may have been placed in foster care, or if the alleged perpetrator is a relative or family friend, there may be an order preventing or limiting further contact with the child. In these cases, the primary question presented to the evaluator may be whether or under what circumstances the child should resume contact with the perpetrator.

However, when allegations of abuse arise in the course of a court-ordered custody evaluation, the questions facing the evaluator grow more complex. The child may have regular contact with the alleged perpetrator. Allegations of abuse may join many other accusations of mistreatment that embittered parties make against each other in the heat of battle. Alternatively, the break-up of the family and the attentive ear of the evaluator may allow abuse that has gone unnoticed or unnamed to be given voice.

Court-ordered evaluations frequently highlight the ways in which intergenerational psychodynamic and interpersonal conflicts can be played out in the courts. The evaluation of a family often vividly depicts the ways in which the legal system can both set the stage for and influence the complex interplay of intrapsychic and interpersonal histories that determine family dramas. When the private life of a family enters the public arena of the court, those surrounding the battle become not only audience to, but participants in, the family's pain. Some of the participation is straightforward; an attorney agrees to represent the interests of one party or another. But sometimes the attorney, too, has multiple motives; she may agree to represent a client in order to promote a particular political, legal, or philosophical position.* Inevitably, as in any human drama, some of the unconscious forces of each of the participants play themselves out in the course of the evaluation.

The facts that constitute the lives of the family sent for assessment are essential in determining the outcome of any evaluation. Ultimately, however, the manifestations of transference, not only in relation to the evaluator, but among the parties, may be even more crucial in analyzing and understanding the conscious and unconscious information that emerges during the evaluation process. In an evaluation in which abuse is either a central or peripheral element, just as in treating an abused child, the clinician must be keenly aware of the dynamic interplay among all of the players in order to guard against being hauled into the battle. Indeed, we often feel a tremendous pull to act—to take sides, to stop listening before the story has been fully revealed, to move quickly and avoid reflection, to assume that the conscious elements of the story take precedence over unconscious dynamics, and to avoid knowing the most painful aspects of a family's life.

This last issue can pose particular difficulties for clinicians whose primary work involves protection of an individual's or family's privacy in order to make space and time for quiet reflection. In addition to the familiar wish to avoid knowing the atrocities that family members inflict on each other in order to protect ourselves from overwhelming affect, we also often must struggle with the wish to help a family avoid a public display of their most private and intimate beings (Bollas & Sundelson, 1995). This may cause special difficulty when the most pertinent information comes from the unconscious communications of one or more of the participants.

Sally

Sally confidently and emphatically described her husband's physical abuse and emotional mistreatment of their 3-year-old daughter, Tillie.

---

*For example, in California there are several cases involving the rights of lesbian parents currently before the courts. Often the attorneys involved have taken these cases to court, not simply for the benefit of the particular family, but for the stated purpose of establishing a legal precedent.

She complained that Tillie had a rash when she returned home from visits to her father because her father refused to rinse Tillie's clothes thoroughly. To support her allegation, she pointed to several small, red spots on Tillie's arm. She had similar complaints about the food Tillie's father prepared, the bedtime stories he read, and the activities he chose. Some of her concerns seemed patently foolish, for example, that he served Tillie bananas without milk, which posed a threat of the child's choking. Others, such as involving Tillie in his own dare-devil athletic pursuits, had more merit. Unfortunately, over the course of the evaluation, as Sally's paranoia became more pronounced, her opinions became more rigidly held, and her distrust of Tillie's father intensified to the point that she could not tolerate any contact at all between Tillie and him. The evaluator felt that Sally's lack of conscious awareness about her own aggressive impulses toward her daughter or her jealousy over the attention Tillie received from her father posed a genuine psychological danger to Tillie.

Knowing that it would likely heighten Sally's paranoia, he nevertheless recommended that until greater emotional stability could be established, Tillie should have only supervised visits with her mother. Understandably, Sally felt that the evaluator had ignored all of the information she had given and that Tillie's father had once again fooled the world into believing that he was a great father. Because of her psychopathology, Sally could not begin to understand or accept the importance of her unconscious communications. In this particular instance, the evaluator was reluctant to make public, that is, to describe explicitly in his report the degree of Sally's emotional fragility. He was concerned that this opinion would lead to Sally's becoming even more entrenched in her position, less amenable to psychotherapy, and therefore less able to assume a full parental role. The evaluator also worried about Tillie's father's lack of empathy for the degree of Sally's anxieties. Although he did not see the father as a malicious man, he feared that the information about Sally's emotional condition would merely confirm the father's belief that Sally's concerns were "crazy." However, the evaluator was able to address these issues, both in the report, and directly with Tillie's father. Fortunately, once the evaluation supported the father's contention that Sally's accusations were unfounded, he could allow himself some curiosity about the motivations for her behavior, which in turn permitted him to be more helpful to Tillie. For the first time, he could consider the possibility that Tillie might benefit from psychotherapy, not merely to undo the damage Sally's "craziness" had inflicted on their daughter, but also to help Tillie with the loss of her mother as a primary attachment figure and to consider his contributions to Tillie's anxieties.

In this case, the evaluation was relatively simple because the relevant transference paradigms were fairly straightforward. Sally's paranoid complaints allowed the father to assign all of the "craziness" in the family to her, without having to confront the real anxieties that his risk-taking behavior caused Tillie. In turn, his dare-devil athletic pursuits provided reality-based concerns for Sally's worries about her daughter's safety. The cast of characters here was small, and the issues of child abuse were fairly easily resolved. In other families, as in the one described below, particularly those involving more players and more interwoven histories, the web of psychodynamic and interpersonal issues is much more difficult to untangle.

Rita and Joy

The battle that brought this family to evaluation was waged not between two warring parents, but between a young woman, Rita, and her parents. After years of struggling to overcome a dangerous and debilitating drug habit, Rita had reached a point in her life when she felt confident about taking over the care of her 6-year-old daughter, Joy. In the course of her recovery, she had settled into a stable relationship and married. She and her new husband, Bill, whom she had met in a drug rehab program, were determined to establish the "normal" family that each of them had missed in their childhoods. Rita's determination to reclaim her child set in motion a process that resulted in the examination and evaluation of the psychodynamics of three generations—Rita, her parents, and her child.

By the age of 12, Rita's life in an upper-middle-class neighborhood had come apart. She attended school only sporadically and showed little regard for any authority that her parents or teachers attempted to exercise over her behavior. By the age of 13, she was regularly prostituting herself to support a drug habit. At the age of 14, she approached her parents for money for an abortion. She did not know or appear to care who the father of the baby might be. Her parents granted her request. Her mother, Mrs. P, had intended to accompany her daughter to the abortion clinic, but neither she nor Rita could remember what had become of that plan.

Joy was born 9 months later; Rita was 15. Over the next few years, Rita bounced in and out of her parents' home, the streets, and drug rehabilitation programs. Most of the time, Joy lived with her grandparents, who had been named her legal guardians, although she had also spent periods of her early life with her mother. Unless they thought Rita was drugged or intoxicated, Mr. and Mrs. P always allowed her contact with Joy, with the stated hope that one day Rita would be able to care for her daughter.

However, following one extended visit with her mother, Joy was discovered to have gonorrhea. This both put a temporary end to Rita's having unsupervised time with her daughter and propelled Rita into a drug-rehabilitation program.

To everyone's amazement Rita did finally succeed in making a life for herself that could accommodate her daughter. As she became more stable, her determination to solidify her relationship with Joy increased. Along with regular visits with Joy at home, Rita made efforts to become involved in Joy's school, to take her to the park, the zoo, and other outings, and to have her spend the night in her home. These arrangements seemed to proceed relatively smoothly, although Mrs. P often complained that Joy was better off at "home" and didn't need to be doing so much with Rita.

However, when Rita and Bill announced their intention to have Joy move into their home, Mrs. P became frantic and immediately contacted the family's attorney. In response, Bill and Rita also hired an attorney. Each side petitioned the court for full legal and physical custody. On the recommendation of the family court mediator, the court appointed an attorney to represent Joy and ordered a psychological evaluation, to address two questions: first, with whom Joy should live, and second, what contact she should have with the other parties?

The Family

While the problem could be stated very simply, the evaluator faced a quite daunting task in attempting to gather, integrate, and analyze the multiple levels of information that would inform the recommendations. The individual and family dynamics that created this conflict and interfered with its resolution had grown more complex and insidious over the course of Rita's childhood, adolescence, and early adulthood. The relationship between Rita and her mother was the locus of tension. Although he was a successful businessman, at home

Mr. P managed conflict by withdrawing; he simply deferred to his wife's judgments and removed himself from the fray, both emotionally and physically. When the battles between Rita and her mother became especially fierce, Mrs. P would take to her bed, claiming that she would likely die of a heart attack within a short time. Only when the animosity reached this pitch would Mr. P intervene—chastising Rita for upsetting her mother.

With the exception of her grandparents, those who knew Joy saw her as a highly immature child who became extremely unpleasant when she didn't get her way. By the end of kindergarten, she had not yet mastered the basic social skills that could enable her to enjoy playing with other children. She couldn't share toys and refused to participate in any game she did not choose. When asked to complete a bit of school work, Joy typically responded that it was too hard, or that she needed more help, or that she didn't understand the directions. When she complained of a stomachache, her teachers gratefully sent her to the principal's office in order to enjoy a break from her incessant whining.

Joy's demands on her grandmother were unrelenting. She frequently refused to leave school unless her grandmother promised to buy her a toy on the way home. Now and then Mrs. P would threaten to leave her at school, which only resulted in Joy's throwing herself on the ground, kicking frenetically, and screaming that everybody hated her and that she would kill herself. Grandmother quickly capitulated to Joy's demand.

Though not obese, Joy was significantly overweight. To some extent this stemmed from her penchant for sweets. Her grandmother attempted to restrict the amount of candy she consumed by hiding the bag of candy and giving Joy only a couple of pieces at a time. Mrs. P frequently forgot where she had hidden the candy, but she usually found only empty bags when she did remember where she had secreted them. During preschool, Joy had refused to eat lunch unless her grandmother brought her food from her favorite fast-food restaurant. The school quickly put a stop to this, only to learn that Joy and her grandmother routinely stopped at that restaurant on the way home as a reward for Joy's good behavior at school.

In general, Mrs. P did not see her relationship to Joy as overly indulgent or infantalizing but, rather, as an understandable and necessary antidote to the excessively harsh and demanding way Rita and Bill treated Joy. She criticized their rigidity, seeing it as an outgrowth of the drug rehabilitation that had successfully enabled them to overcome their addictions. However, Mrs. P appreciated this program's salvaging her daughter's life, which she had not been able to do despite years of trying.

When Rita was growing up, Mr. and Mrs. P had regularly bailed her out of scrapes at school and in the neighborhood; they could see nothing in her behavior other than an adolescent rebellion. Mrs. P now frequently reminded Rita that they had tried to be good parents, even though Rita had always been a difficult child. In contrast to her daughter, Mrs. P found Joy a very easy child to raise. She felt that Rita often mistakenly saw herself in Joy, which led her to use unnecessarily harsh disciplinary tactics. Mrs. P believed strongly that the methods used to treat adult drug addicts should not be used for raising young children. When Joy did not meet Rita and Bill's expectations, they usually disciplined her by having her stand ramrod straight, facing the wall, for several minutes at time. Mrs. P felt this bordered on child abuse. She found her method of rewarding Joy with a small bit of candy or a trinket much more effective.

From Mrs. P's perspective, children could be raised with either rewards or punishments: She just happened to be more comfortable with rewards, while Rita and Bill preferred punishments. Mrs. P frequently told them that she felt they abused Joy. Indeed, on one occasion Mrs. P had called Child Protective Services after Joy reported that Bill had hit her with a wooden spoon. The investigation had not resulted in any action against Bill or Rita except a recommendation that they enroll in parenting classes.

Bill and Rita did subscribe to a philosophy akin to "spare the rod and spoil the child." They pointed to Joy's behavior as evidence for the correctness of their position. Bill had no regrets about having spanked Joy; this seemed to him a perfectly reasonable punishment for Joy's stealing and eating an entire box of candy. Both he and Rita felt strongly that the erratic discipline that they had received as children had contributed to their drug abuse. They saw Joy's greediness as addictive behavior, which left them terrified, particularly because Mrs. P seemed so oblivious to her contribution to either Rita's or Joy's problems.

They felt that Joy's behavior changed dramatically in their home. After an initial period of testing limits, she behaved much more maturely; the whining stopped, and Joy readily complied with expectations. They attributed this transformation to their policy of quickly and firmly punishing any misbehavior rather than waiting for it to worsen. Joy was expected to follow the rules without complaint. At the first sign of protest, she went to the wall. They were pleased that Joy rarely whined or complained more than once or twice and only at the beginning of a visit.

Bill and Rita had enrolled in the parenting class because they felt it would help them in their efforts to gain custody of Joy. They found some of the information useful, but they felt that the philosophy of parenting focused too much on understanding the child's feelings and not enough on respecting authority.

The Therapists

From very early in Rita's childhood, Mr. and Mrs. P had consulted a number of therapists. According to Rita, her mother just "chewed them up and spit them out." According to Mrs. P, most of them "weren't worth a sack of beans." At the time of the evaluation, Rita and Bill were involved in family counseling and Joy was in individual psychotherapy.

The family therapist, Ms. M, was extremely sympathetic to Rita and Bill's wish to bring their family together. She was appalled by Rita's stories of a grim childhood characterized by her mother's vicious verbal assaults and occasional physical attacks with a belt or hairbrush. Rita described feeling completely unprotected because of her father's passivity in the face of these outbursts and her mother's periodic threats of an impending heart attack. At these times, Mr. P had advised Rita to follow his lead and simply learn to ignore her. For Rita this represented an intolerable submission, as well as threatening the loss of the most intense contact she had with her mother.

Ms. M found Rita and Bill's description of Mrs. P's relationship with Joy equally upsetting. In addition to her concern that Joy was trapped in an infantalized position in order to avoid her grandmother's wrath, Mrs. P's continuing to bathe, dress, and sleep with this 6-year-old girl, raised questions in her mind about the sexualized nature of their relationship. When Rita and Bill told her that Joy was unable to fall asleep without masturbating, the family therapist's concerns deepened. Although Joy had never said, or otherwise indicated, that either grandparent touched her genitals other than in bathing her, the family counselor felt that she was, at the very least, being overstimulated by the sleeping and bathing arrangements. The significance of her concerns prompted her to write a letter, via Rita and Bill's attorney, urging the court to award full custody of Joy to Rita and to act as swiftly as possible.

Joy had been referred by her school to Ms. S for individual psychotherapy about 6 months prior to the evaluation. Ms. S had declined requests to write to the court on behalf of either Rita's or Mr. and Mrs. P's position. While this left each party somewhat skeptical of her professional judgment, she remained firmly convinced that she could not maintain the neutrality necessary for her work with Joy if she were forced to take a stance about Joy's living arrangements. In the letter that she did write to the court, she asked that any recommendations be resolved through the evaluation process, which she promised to support.

Ms. S had been aware of Joy's masturbatory behavior, which, according to her records, Mrs. P had noted from early in Joy's life. In her opinion, Joy's compulsive masturbation stemmed primarily from two sources: first, as a predictable consequence of the presumed sexual abuse Joy had suffered, which resulted in her contracting gonorrhea, and second, as a means of self-comfort that had developed in the chaos and lack of reliable care that had permeated Joy's early life. She shared Ms. M's concerns about the sleeping and bathing arrangements and made some suggestions to all of the adults about ways they could help Joy with this as well as other symptoms. However, she expected that Joy's symptoms, some of which had begun to abate prior to the court battle, would intensify over the course of the evaluation.

From her perspective, Joy appeared to be deeply attached to both her mother and her grandmother and gravely troubled by their ongoing battles. She felt that Mrs. P's anxiety about losing Joy had made it more difficult for her to contain her negative feelings about Rita. She expressed concern that Joy frequently served as audience for her grandmother's diatribes against her mother. Ms. S felt that the severe limitations both women brought to parenting hid some positive attributes each had to offer Joy.

She felt that Mrs. P's indulgence and infantilization easily masked the patience this woman showed when Joy struggled to maintain control of her behavior or meet the demands of school. She offered too much food too readily, but she did so, at least partially, from her recognition of Joy's pervasive sense of deprivation and loss. However, she maintained this behavior partly because of her great investment in seeing Joy's difficulties arising from Rita's abandonment rather than from her own relationship with her granddaughter.

Ms. S agreed that Joy's behavior had matured strikingly during the time she spent with Rita and Bill. However, she felt that this reflected both her wariness of their anger and a compliance with external demands rather than demonstrating significant internal shifts. She thought that Bill and Rita espoused an attitude toward parenting somewhat more rigid in theory than in practice. Although they sometimes disciplined Joy rather harshly, they also devoted enormous energy to activities that she enjoyed, including sports, which they hoped would have the added benefit of helping her to reduce her weight. By and large, their expectations of Joy were reasonable and their reluctance to tolerate Joy's symptomatic behavior was more in keeping with the demands placed on her at school. Ms. S felt that they had begun to make some rudimentary distinctions between bribing and rewarding and between appropriately firm and overly harsh punishments that might eventually give them more tools for parenting Joy.

The Attorneys

Because of the court proceedings, the family had acquired yet another level of experts—the attorneys who would interpret, advise, and help them make their way through the legal system. Like the therapists, each brought a particular bias to the work and added to the complexity of the family's dynamics.

The attorney representing Joy's grandparents was an old friend and colleague of Mr. P who took a stance of bemused detachment toward the evaluation. Mr. W expected the court to have little success in controlling Mrs. P's behavior, regardless of the outcome of the evaluation. Over the years, he had been called in numerous times to intervene with school authorities or the justice system to keep Rita out of juvenile hall. He had developed a sympathetic respect for her tenacious struggles to make a life for herself, but he didn't like her. He found Rita as abrasive and self-centered as her mother. In his opinion, the two of them would always need something to fight about—this round just happened to be over Joy.

Ms. A, the attorney representing Rita and Bill had a reputation for battling ferociously for her clients. She most frequently represented parents in their efforts to regain custody of their children. Philosophically, politically, and legally she was committed to the sanctity of family bonds and believed that, except under the most extreme circumstances, children belonged with their parents. She made convincing arguments about the emotional suffering of adopted children who spent much of their lives searching for their biological parents.

Generally, she was skeptical of arguments in favor of protecting a child's attachment to a substitute parent. She used any evidence of psychopathology in that relationship to bolster her arguments, and the relationship between Joy and her grandmother provided her with an abundance of ammunition.

The most recent addition to the cast of characters was Joy's court-appointed attorney, Mr. B, who frequently represented foster parents in their efforts either to adopt or maintain contact with a child who had initially been placed with them for temporary care. Although he represented different legal positions, philosophically he leaned toward protecting a child's emotional bond to a parent or parent substitute over privileging the biological relationship between parent and child.

By the end of the evaluation, he had been so inundated with enraged and abusive phone calls and materials from both parties that he had found himself wondering if there might not be an option that didn't include either Joy's mother or her grandparents! The pleasant cooperation which had characterized his initial contacts with Rita and Bill and Mr. and Mrs. P had disintegrated relatively quickly into hostility on both fronts. When they could agree on nothing else, Rita and her mother concurred that Mr. B had no business in their lives and no reason to assume that he could know better than her family how Joy should be raised.

Mr. B was most impressed with the meanness permeating Rita and Mrs. P's descriptions of each other. He worried that both relied on the admittedly ample evidence from each side to blame the other for Joy's difficulties. Neither of them seemed inclined to assume responsibility for the potential negative effects of her behavior on Joy. Although Rita readily acknowledged that Joy had suffered tremendously as a result of her active drug addiction, she attributed Joy's present difficulties almost exclusively to Mrs. P's influence. For her part, Mrs. P accepted only that any mistakes she had made as a parent would have been made by anyone trying to raise a child as difficult as Rita.

Despite his irritation, Mr. B felt that much of this grandmother's defensiveness stemmed from her barely conscious awareness of the ways in which she had failed Rita and her attempts at reparation through her relationship with Joy. His concern about Rita focused on her apparent need to "cure" Joy in order to prove herself a better mother than Mrs. P. While less pathological parenting would certainly benefit Joy, he worried that Rita's emphasis on obedience and appropriate behavior had more to do with seeing herself as a good parent than on promoting Joy's emotional health.

The Evaluation

The evaluator's contacts with this family and the supporting characters extended over several months. As is so often the case, the evaluation uncovered more ambiguities than certainties. The unconsciously shared meanings and psychopathologies of Joy's immediate and extended family were so intertwined that separating them even for the purpose of discussion was difficult. That they could ever be fully disentangled in Joy's actual life seemed improbable. However, the court asked that all the available information be considered in addressing two questions: first, with whom Joy should live, and second, what contact should she have with the other parties?

Consideration of the People and Issues

Joy had contracted gonorrhea early in her life, presumably while in Rita's care. Although the incubation period for this infection did not preclude Joy's having been sexually abused while in the care of her grandparents, this possibility had never been raised by any of the parties. The most likely explanation for Joy's contracting gonorrhea lay in Rita's drug addiction—she had either offered her daughter as a sexual object in exchange for drugs/money, or because of a drug-induced stupor, she had been unable to protect Joy from sexual exploitation by one or more of her many contacts.

Though Rita's behavioral patterns from preadolescence through young adulthood resembled those commonly seen in children who have been sexually abused, there were no allegations of or allusions to familial sexual abuse in any of Rita's records or in the evaluation interviews. However, her family's failure to protect her had resulted in Rita's prostituting herself, that is, making herself available for sexual exploitation as a young adolescent. Clearly, there had been two children involved in these horrible circumstances—Rita was a drug-addicted child, just 15 years old when she gave birth to Joy. Six years later—clean and sober—she wanted to assume the role of a responsible adult.

Although Mr. P's presence in the family was greatly overshadowed by his wife and daughter, in his quiet way, he appeared to provide a stabilizing force for Joy. Their relationship, based on mutual affection, appeared to be nestled quietly between Mrs. P's histrionics and Rita's rage. On the one hand, Joy seemed to have learned from her grandfather what her mother could not, namely, that sometimes much can be gained from just staying out of the way. On the other hand, Mr. P had emotionally abandoned Rita in the face of his wife's rages. He would very likely repeat this behavior if Joy's efforts to break the symbiotic tie to her grandmother engendered similar behavior toward Joy.

All of the available evidence suggested that Mrs. P could not easily support or tolerate Joy's beginning attempts at separation. The hostile symbiosis between Mrs. P and Joy successfully contained the rage that each unconsciously expected could destroy their relationship. There were abundant reasons to recommend that Mr. and Mrs. P's guardianship be terminated. Mrs. P was a volatile woman who destroyed relationships as quickly as she made them. Joy regularly witnessed her grandmother's tirades against family, friends, teachers, or salespeople, in short, anyone whose behavior displeased her at any moment. Neither Rita's history nor current psychological status argued well for Mr. and Mrs. P's successful parenting. Of course, parental influence is only one of many factors that contribute to personality, and, in many cases, grandparents enjoy more success raising their grandchildren than they did raising their children. Nevertheless, the profoundly pathological relationship between Joy and her grandmother argued strenuously against having Mr. and Mrs. P continue in a parenting role.

However, Joy was a fragile child who had endured multiple disruptions and losses early in her life. Although she was attached to both Rita and Mrs. P, her grandmother was her primary psychological parent. Removing Joy from her grandparents' care would not be without negative psychological consequences. First it would constitute a painful loss of the one person who, however flawed, had been most consistent in her life. Secondly, a recommendation favoring Rita would probably constitute such a narcissistic injury to Mrs. P that she might withdraw entirely from Joy just at the time Joy needed her help and support in making the transition to her mother's care.

Therefore, the primary argument for extending the grandparents' guardianship would be negative, that is, to avoid the loss of a pathological relationship, rather than to maintain or support a healthy relationship. Secondarily, one had to consider the possibility of keeping Joy with her grandparents in order to avoid entrusting her to her mother's care.

The stress of the evaluation had demonstrated the fragility of both Rita's and Bill's impulse control. Although they had tried valiantly to maintain a cooperative and cordial relationship to Joy's attorney and the evaluator, their demeanor gradually settled into one of "Either you're with me or you're against me." This stance allowed for little questioning of their motivations or behavior without arousing suspiciousness and defensive hostility. Indeed, Bill's knowledge that his spanking Joy risked losing their custody bid had not prevented his hitting her under the virtual gaze of the court, three attorneys, two therapists, and an evaluator, let alone his mother-in-law, whose ruthlessness in battle he and Rita knew all too well!

Even if Rita had agreed in principle that Joy's behavior justified a spanking, her potential willingness to sabotage the custody battle raised serious questions about her abilities to ascertain the nuances of others' expectations and the consequences of her behavior. Further, Rita's support of this spanking raised the question of how she would react if Bill's physical punishments became even more harsh. Equally important, it suggested significant limitations in Rita's capacity to understand and empathize with the complex emotional motivations for Joy's behavior. Again, granting that Joy's taking a box of candy without permission and consuming its entire contents might exceed the bounds of acceptable behavior, Bill's response (supported by Rita) did not appear, in either word nor deed, to take into account the possibility that Joy was so anxious about losing one or more of the people she loved most in the world that she felt compelled to gobble up everything in sight as a profound, though unconscious, defense against an unbearable emptiness.

Thus, paradoxically, although it appeared that Rita and Bill favored and fostered Joy's maturation and independence (in contrast to Mrs. P's infantilization of her), they actually, although unconsciously, saw Joy's behavior as a vehicle reflecting their own successes or failures rather than recognizing her actions as expressions of her own internal processes. Interestingly, this demonstrated an unconsciously shared perspective between Mrs. P and Rita, namely, that children were responsible for their failures, whereas parents were responsible for children's successes. So, while superficially it appeared as if Rita could recognize and support Joy's developmental needs to establish herself as a separate and autonomous being, the motivation for her focus on Joy's independence was actually self-referential—Rita needed to see herself as a good mother, which required that Joy behave in the particular ways that Rita had defined as demonstrating parental success.

To some extent all parents may look to their children's behavior as a measure of their successes or failures in parenting. However there is a fundamental distinction between viewing a child's actions solely as a reflection or extension of the parent(s)' behavior, attitudes, or personality and seeing aspects of parental influences represented in a child's uniquely evolving character. Rita, like her own mother, showed little capacity to consider Joy's behavior as internally motivated. For Rita, Joy's infantile behavior represented her connection to Mrs. P, while independence and maturity represented a connection to her. This made Joy's regressions intolerable, for Rita saw them as evidence of Joy slipping away from her. It was extremely difficult for Rita to consider the fluctuations in Joy's behavior as manifestations of her internal states, separate from her relationship to either her mother or her grandmother.

Thus, while placement with Rita might be problematic for a number of reasons, Rita's inability to grant Joy a separate existence posed a great threat to Joy's healthy development. Because Rita's stated objective was to foster independence, helping her to see the ways in which she did not fully differentiate her own needs, motivations, or behavior from Joy's would likely pose a formidable task.

Although Bill and Rita had jointly retained Ms. A in their efforts to gain custody of Joy, Bill actually was not a party to the case. He had no relationship to Joy that allowed him legal standing in the proceedings; he was neither Joy's biological nor adoptive parent. The judge had denied his petition for *de facto* parent status* on the grounds that his interests were sufficiently congruent with Rita's such that no

---

*"*De facto* parent" is a legal term that refers to an adult's having stood in parental relationship to a child by virtue of having performed the usual functions of a parent on a regular and important basis. "Psychological parent" refers to the person(s) whom the child relates to as if a parent. In other words, the child's behavior toward that person reflects that person's parental status in the child's internal world. For most children, the biological, legal, and psychological parent are one and the same. However, the relationships represented by these sometimes overlapping terms can become both very confused and important in custody battles.

separate representation was necessary and that his status as a *de facto* parent was entirely contingent on his relationship to Rita. Despite his lack of a legal relationship to Joy, Bill was an integral part of the psychological landscape surrounding the relationship between Joy and Rita. Bill did appear to have a stabilizing influence on both Rita and Joy; his quick disciplinary actions provided a striking contrast to Rita's tendency to assault Joy verbally. While Rita readily described her philosophy of firm, reasonable behavioral consequences, she easily got pulled into angry recriminations in the face of Joy's demands and regression. Bill's responses tended to be more simple and straightforward. However, this focus on behavior and consequences resulted in a rather robotic quality to his relationship with Joy. Pleasurable activities, such as a trip to the zoo or playing a game, seemed to be offered only as a reward for good behavior rather than for fun! Any mutual enjoyment or satisfaction appeared to be of only secondary importance—bedtime stories encouraged children to read; team sports provided exercise and lessons in cooperation; outings offered educational opportunities.

In Bill's world, there seemed to be little chance to eat a piece of candy just for the sheer pleasure it offered. Although Bill had spanked Joy for eating the entire box of candy, having any treat that one had not earned could also prompt a punishment, though perhaps not one so harsh. The voices of Bill's inner world appeared to speak a demanding and critical language which, for much of his life, had been softened by drugs. In his efforts to maintain his recovery from addiction, Bill struggled to modulate his own impulses with an unyielding focus on reasonable and "fair" behavior. The motivations underlying behavior held little interest for him; the distinctions between conscious and unconscious, between rational and irrational, had no meaning; outcome alone counted. Bill took pride and comfort in his uncomplicated attitude toward parenting—reward behavior you want, and punish behavior you don't.

Ms. A, Rita and Bill's attorney aptly put forward their desire for a world uncomplicated by ambiguity. If she saw any merit in Mr. and Mrs. P's case or any value in Joy's relationship to her grandparents, she kept that view entirely to herself. Consciously, they chose someone whose views closely reflected their own. Their behavior and attitudes suggested that an unconscious wish to avoid the anxiety raised when they could not so easily split the world into good and bad also motivated their choice of attorneys.

The questions and uncertainties raised by the evaluator, Mr. B, and Joy's therapist all engendered considerable anxiety in Rita and Bill. A suggestion that Joy might enjoy some aspects of her relationship to her grandparents seemed to suggest that Mr. and Mrs. P were good and they were bad. Rita tried to appreciate Joy's attachment to Mr. and Mrs. P, but her fear and rage at them made it exceedingly difficult for her to support Joy's love for them. (Of course, Mrs. P's continual quiet undermining of Rita along with her frequent rages at Rita for being an ungrateful daughter and an unfit mother did not help.) Rita and Bill tended to hear Joy's therapist's insistence on the importance of Joy's relationship to both them and her grandparents as a rather cowardly means of supporting the grandparents' position over theirs.

Perhaps because they accurately viewed Mr. B as the person charged with speaking for Joy in the legal proceedings, their behavior with him most vividly demonstrated their difficulty in tolerating ambivalence in a relationship. Their initial pleasant and deferential cooperation with Mr. B changed to rage at the moment he explained to Rita and Bill that he needed to meet with Joy in addition to hearing their view of what would be in Joy's best interests. They understood this as a statement that he disbelieved or disagreed with them, as well as a challenge to the parental authority they so desperately wanted to assert. They had simply assumed that Mr. B would join in the fight for the correctness of their position.

Both Mr. B and Ms. S recognized that the barrage of attacks and counterattacks swirling around them stemmed from their unwillingness to take sides in the battle. What they saw as a neutral stance, Rita and Mrs. P each saw as granting validity to the other's position. Because both Rita and Mrs. P viewed the world in black and white terms, conceding any point meant losing the entire argument, which meant that each felt that she absolutely must win Mr. B's allegiance. If gentle persuasion didn't work, both were quite relentless in their conscious and unconscious attempts to pound him into submission.

Mr. B confessed that he had, many times, found himself searching for legitimate reasons for removing himself from this case. When it occurred to him that he actually had an option that Joy did not have, his appreciation for her emotional torment deepened. Although she was profoundly attached to both her mother and grandmother, their struggles made it impossible for her to love either of them fully. Because of their own limitations and fears, they had constructed her world to mean that loving one person meant not loving another. This left Joy trapped in an untenable limbo.

Possible Custody Arrangements

The very toxic relationships Joy had available to her within her family raised the consideration of foster care as a potentially viable alternative. Although neither of the two obvious choices was inviting, the evaluator eliminated foster care as a third possibility on a number of grounds. First, there were no other family members available to step in as foster parents, which would mean placing Joy with strangers. She had already suffered numerous losses, and her ties to her family were profound, though exceedingly troubled. Moving her outside of her family would assuredly subject her to two stressful losses, possibly more, if she became attached to and then removed from a family. Second, the foster care system offers no guarantees of a stable long-term placement, and, unfortunately, foster homes are not always safe; foster placement introduced a risk of physical, emotional, or sexual harm. Third, legally required consideration of family reunification would require Joy's having ongoing, even if limited, contact with her mother or grandmother or both. This would merely move the current conflict to a new arena and introduce more players and greater complexity. In addition, foster parents who had to endure significant contact with either Rita or Mrs. P might well move Joy along rather than suffer their aggression and insults. Fourth, a recommendation for temporary foster placement would set in motion a protracted legal process, with all of its accompanying uncertainties and animosities. Although dire, Joy's circumstances were unlikely to warrant a case for the termination of either Rita's or Mr. and Mrs. P's legal/parental rights. Therefore, even if foster care presented a temporary solution, the benefits of removing Joy from her family battleground did not outweigh the attendant risks.

Joy's continuing to live with her grandparents offered little hope for her escape from the emotional morass in which she lived. Over the course of raising Rita and Joy, Mrs. P had shown no interest in examining her attitudes, behavior, or relationships. Although the family had consulted with many competent therapists, nothing substantial had changed. While Mr. B intuited that Mrs. P might have some vague awareness of her negative impact on Rita, she showed little inclination toward finding more positive ways of relating to her daughter. Superficially, Mrs. P's relationship with Joy seemed different from her relationship to Rita. She adored, indulged, and catered to Joy. However, Joy was allowed no separate self; she remained pathologically attached to an infantile relationship with her grandmother. She paid the price of a symbiotic attachment in order to avoid her grandmother's wrath; she ordered her grandmother about, rather than risking autonomous steps that left her grandmother behind. Controlling hostility and regression substituted for assertion and independence.

However, moving Joy into Rita and Bill's care also posed very serious threats to her physical and emotional well-being. Bill and Rita were newly recovering addicts whose hold on a clean and sober life would be tested by full-time parenthood. However, the prime danger for Joy lay in her attempting both to preserve her relationships with them and to avoid physical or verbal assaults by unconsciously setting aside the very essence of her being. Along with low self-esteem, Joy had a very tenuous relationship to her self—her separate and unique feelings, needs, and desires. Bill's and Rita's need for conformity, validation, and relationships unchallenged by difference or disagreement threatened to force Joy into a position of developing a false self—a superficially coherent personality organization masking a profound emptiness and affective impoverishment.

Both courses of action posed very great risks. Like Mr. B, Joy's attorney, the evaluator recognized the wish to leave this case behind as a reflection of Joy's dilemma and helplessness. The desire simply to create new parents for Joy represented the wish to destroy history, to give her a better life than she had lived. The evaluator, like Joy, could not escape two extremely problematic alternatives.

The Recommendation

The evaluator recommended, with grave reservations, that Joy live with her mother and Bill. As individuals and as a couple Rita and Bill had struggled against overwhelming odds to gain control of their addictions and lead the lives of respectable citizens. While much in their behavior pointed to their accommodation to externally generated standards rather than to a successful integration of internally generated change, the center did seem to be holding. The stress of the evaluation had shown the cracks in their defensive organizations, but it had not led to irreparable fractures; by neither resuming drug use nor running from the evaluation, they demonstrated an increased capacity to tolerate both frustration and anxiety. Bill had spanked Joy in a controlled, purposeful manner, rather than in a terrifyingly impulsive rage; he regretted having to resort to corporal punishment but simply did not see a spanking as falling outside the bounds of reasonable parental behavior. He and Rita agreed that Rita's verbal rages probably frightened Joy more.

The recommendation to grant custody to Rita was contingent upon their moving to a different family therapist. The evaluator acknowledged the importance of their work with Ms. M, agreeing that without her support and encouragement they might not have had the confidence to pursue their fight for Joy. They drew strength from her unwavering, positive view of them as individuals and parents. However, the same qualities and attitudes that had sustained them in their battle now held the possibility of interfering with their attempts to establish their fervently desired "normal" family with three clearly demarcated generations, in which grandparents deferred to the primacy and authority of the parent–child relationship, and the parents respected the unique bond between grandparents and grandchild.

The success of this recommendation rested largely on Rita's and Bill's capacity to help Joy sustain a relationship with her grandparents in the face of Mrs. P's anticipated onslaughts. Although Ms. M and Mrs. P had never met, they openly disliked and disrespected what they knew of each other; this did not leave Ms. M in a viable position for helping Rita and Bill to navigate the treacherous waters that lay ahead. Whether or not the new family therapist elected to have contact with Mr. and Mrs. P, a genuine appreciation for their importance in Joy's life, as well as in Rita's, would be essential for helping this family to reorganize in ways that allowed for less pathological interactions.

In the summary,* the evaluator discussed the inherent limitations of the family's emotional resources and the difficulties of attempting to resolve complex family problems through the courts. The very serious psychopathology in Joy's family minimized the chances of creating a truly healthy environment for her. Even if all of the players

---

*The summary also included specific recommendations for Joy's living arrangements, school placement, continuation in individual therapy, and mechanisms for visits with her grandparents that are not pertinent to this discussion.

followed the rules laid down by the court, it seemed likely that they would participate by acting according to the letter, rather than the spirit of the law.

While planning and hoping for the best, the evaluator feared that the individual psychopathologies of this family were so deeply ingrained and enmeshed that these people would be unable to move beyond their crippling family drama, even to save the life of a child whom all of the adults, in some way, loved and cared for. Like the artist who must tailor his art to the attributes of the available materials (Caper, 1996), we must accept the inherent limitations on our wishes to create a supportive, nurturing, loving family for each child we encounter. Sometimes the best we can do is point the "actors" in the drama in the right direction and offer them the tools to work toward giving their children the very great gift of a "good enough" environment.

Conclusion

In the preceding chapters, I have attempted to address many of the complex factors involved in comprehending and treating children who have been emotionally, physically, or sexually abused. To understand fully a child who comes to us for help, we must consider the individual child within her or his particular environment, making careful note of the interplay between internal and external influences. We consider the child and the abuse she or he suffered with attention to developmental expectations and the ways in which that abuse may have derailed the neurobiological substrata of behavior. We consider her or his symptoms both as windows into these underlying processes and as expressions of personal meaning.

When children either disclose abuse or fail to do so, we understand that their memory of abuse may not be accessible to them, or at least not in a way that allows them to talk about it. We also appreciate the complex ideas and feelings that inhibit them from sharing their experiences with us, even when their memories are accessible. I have tried to elucidate the reasons for and meanings of the symptom clusters we typically associate with abuse, attending particularly to the resistance toward accepting the internal aspects of abusive experiences. This helps to clarify the importance of language in our work with abused children and the paradoxes that beset us when we attempt to put words to events that are monstrous and unspeakable.

Abused children have profound and powerful effects on the people around them. By understanding how they may unconsciously induce others to experience or act on their feelings, we increase the effectiveness of our attempts to assist others who work with them. Particularly in our work with their parents, and substitute parents we must give careful attention to the psychological effects on those entrusted with the care of an abused child. Finally, I have tried to demonstrate that the effects of abuse do not always show themselves directly but may, instead, be perpetuated in unexpected but insidious ways.

This brief summary should serve to remind us of how very much abused children need from us. I hope that the reader takes from this volume an appreciation of the complex demands psychoanalytic psychotherapy makes on child and therapist alike. Further, I hope it will assist those who work with abused children by contributing to their knowledge, their skills, and their capacity to sit quietly with another.

As I began this book, I first heard of the case of two children who had recently been removed from the care of their mother, whose multiple drug addictions had made it impossible for her to care for them. The children had suffered years of neglect and physical abuse; Amber, the 9-year-old girl, had been diagnosed with genital warts. Shortly after their placement with maternal relatives, the children began psychotherapy.

Amber's therapist described her as the quietest child he had ever met. She never spoke unless spoken to. The therapist's questions were followed by pauses extending over several minutes with only monosyllabic responses punctuating the silence. This child showed her intelligence solely in the consistent winning strategies she brought to board games. The therapist never worried about whether to let Amber win; she always did.

Weeks of therapy stretched into months. The therapist sometimes felt as if each session lasted a week; so little seemed to pass between them. Yet, the pauses after comments or questions seemed gradually a little shorter, and Amber sometimes responded with two or three words instead of one. As the weekly meetings moved through the first and into the second year of therapy, Amber occasionally offered an unprompted comment and sometimes selected from among the art materials to make a spontaneous, but unnarrated, project.

About 2½ years after beginning therapy, during the silence with which Amber started each session, she gathered paper, glue, scissors, and markers, and then announced that she intended to make a pop-up book, which she had occasionally done before. The therapist commented that the drawings seemed particularly interesting and, as he had done before, wondered whether there was a story that went with the pictures. Amber looked at him quizzically, then cut a small page from a larger piece of paper and silently began writing. When she filled up the first page, she painstakingly cut another, filled it with writing, cut another, and in this fashion finished a story several pages long.

In words and drawings, Amber told the story of children who happily picked cherries from a tree until the people who owned the tree moved away. Some old, mean people moved in and would no longer allow the children to eat the cherries. The children didn't know what to do until they decided to get their own tree so they would always have enough cherries.

Amber seemed as surprised as her therapist at what she had created. As they worked together to fashion a special binding for her book, he asked her about the process of writing—whether she had written the story as she went along or whether it came to her all at once. She said it just came out. He suggested that perhaps her story had been waiting a very long time to be told and that she must have many more stories to tell. Amber smiled shyly.

I heard this chapter in Amber's story as my writing of this book drew to a close. In the time since I first heard about Amber, I have spent many hours trying to address the complex feelings and ideas that both children and their therapists face in trying to mitigate the effects of abuse. Amber, too, has spent many hours in this endeavor; her brief story poignantly captures the limitations and the promises of this process.

References

Ainsworth, M. D., Blehar, M., Waters, E., & Wall, S. (1978). *Patterns of Attachment*. Hillsdale, NJ: Erlbaum.

Amini, F., Lewis, T., Lannon, R., Louie, A., Baumbacher, G., McGuinness, T., & Schiff, E. Z. (1996). Affect, Attachment, Memory: Contributions toward Psychobiologic Integration. *Psychiatry, 59*, 213–239.

Ashworth, C. S., Fargason, C. A., Jr., & Fountain, K. (1995). Impact of Patient History on Residents' Evaluation of Child Sexual Abuse. *Child Abuse and Neglect, 19*(8), 943–951.

Bays, J., & Chadwick, D. (1993). Medical Diagnosis of the Sexually Abused Child. *Child Abuse and Neglect, 17*, 91–110.

Beck, J. C., & van der Kolk, B. (1987). Reports of Childhood Incest and Current Behavior of Chronically Hospitalized Psychotic Women. *American Journal of Psychiatry, 144*(11), 1474–1476.

Beebe, B., & Lachman, F. (1992). The Contribution of Mother–Infant Mutual Influence to the Origins of Self- and Object Representations. In N. Skolnick & S. Warshaw (Eds.), *Relational Perspectives in Psychoanalysis*. (pp. 83–117). Hillsdale, NJ: Analytic Press.

Benedek, T. (1959). Parenthood as a Developmental Phase: A Contribution to the Libido Theory. *Journal of the American Psychoanalytic Association* 7:389–417.

Birch, M. (1998). Through a Glass Darkly: Questions about Truth and Memory. *Psychoanalytic Psychology, 15*, 34–48.

Birch, M. (1994, April). *Rock-A-Bye Baby: Ordinary Maternal Hate*. Paper presented at the annual meeting of the American Psychological Association, Washington, DC.

Bollas, C., & Sundelson, D. (1995). *The New Informants: The Betrayal of*

Confidentiality in Psychoanalysis and Psychotherapy. Northvale, NJ: Jason Aronson.

Bowlby, J. (1973). *Attachment and Loss: Vol. 2. Separation, Anxiety, and Anger*. New York: Basic Books.

Bowlby, J. (1980). *Attachment and Loss: Vol. 3. Loss, Sadness and Depression*. New York: Basic Books.

Brazelton, T. B., Koslowski, B., & Main, M. (1974). The Early Mother–Infant Interaction. In M. Lewis & L. Rosenblum (Eds.), *The Effect of the Infant on Its Caregiver* (pp. 49–77). New York: Wiley.

Breiner, S. J. (1990). *Slaughter of the Innocents: Child Abuse through the Ages and Today*. New York: Plenum Press.

Bremner, J. D., Krystal, J. H., Charney, D. S., & Southwick, S. M. (1996). Neural Mechanisms in Dissociative Amnesia for Childhood Abuse: Relevance to the Current Controversy Surrounding the "False Memory Syndrome." *American Journal of Psychiatry, 153*(7), 71–82.

Bromberg, P. M. (1996). Hysteria, Dissociation, and Cure. *Psychoanalytic Dialogues, 6*(1), 55–71.

Brown, L. S. (1991). Not Outside the Range: One Feminist Perspective on Psychic Trauma. *American Imago, 48*(1), 119–133.

Burland, J. A. (1994). Splitting as a Consequence of Severe Abuse in Childhood. *Psychiatric Clinics of North America, 17*(4), 731–742.

Call, J. D. (1984). From Early Patterns of Communication to the Grammar of Experience and Syntax in Infancy. In J. D. Call, E. Galenson, & R. L. Tyson (Eds.), *Frontiers of Infant Psychiatry* (Vol. 2, pp. 15–29). New York: Basic Books.

Caper, R. (1996). Play, Experimentation and Creativity. *International Journal of Psycho-Analysis, 77*, 859–869.

Carlin, A. S., Kemper, K., Ward, N. G., Sowell, H., Gustafson, B., & Stevens, N. (1994). The Effect of Differences in Objective and Subjective Definitions of Childhood Physical Abuse on Estimates of Its Incidence and Relationship to Psychopathology. *Child Abuse and Neglect, 18*(5), 393–399.

Cath, S. H., Gurwitt, A. R., & Ross, J. M. (Eds.) (1982). *Father and Child: Developmental and Clinical Perspectives*. Boston: Little, Brown.

Ceci, S. J., Huffman, M. L. C., Smith, E., & Loftus, E. F. (1994). Repeatedly Thinking about a Non-Event: Source Misattributions among Preschoolers. In K. Pezdek & W. P. Banks (Eds.), *The Recovered Memory/False Memory Debate* (pp. 225–244). San Diego: Academic Press.

Ceci, S. J., Loftus, E. F., Leichtman, M. D., & Bruck, M. (1994). The Possible Role of Source Misattributions in the Creation of False Beliefs among Preschoolers. *International Journal of Clinical and Experimental Hypnosis, 42*(4), 304–320.

Chodorow, N. (1978). *Reproduction of Mothering: Psychoanalysis and the Sociology of Gender*. Berkeley: University of California Press.

Chused, J. (1991). The Evocative Power of Enactments. *Journal of the American Psychoanalytic Association, 39*, 615–639.

Coen, C. W. (Ed.). (1985). *Functions of the Brain*. Oxford: Clarendon Press.

Cohen, Y. (1988). The "Golden Fantasy" and Countertransference: Residential Treatment of the Abused Child. *Psychoanalytic Study of the Child, 43*, 337–350.

Conte, J. R. (1995). Assessment of Children Who May Have Been Abused: The Real World Context. In T. Ney (Ed.), *True and False Allegations of Child Sexual Abuse* (pp. 290–302). New York: Brunner/Mazel.

Coppolillo, H. P. (1987). *Psychodynamic Psychotherapy of Children: An Introduction to the Art and the Techniques*. Madison, CT: International Universities Press.

Crothers, D. (1995). Vicarious Traumatization in the Work with Survivors of Childhood Trauma. *Journal of Psychosocial Nursing, 33*, 9–13.

Davies, J. M., & Frawley, M. G. (1991a). Dissociative Processes and Transference–Countertransference Paradigms in the Psychoanalytically Oriented Treatment of Adult Survivors of Childhood Sexual Abuse. *Psychoanalytic Dialogues, 2*(1), 5–36.

DeAngelis, T. (1997, June) When Children Don't Bond with Parents: Psychologists Are Providing a Controversial Treatment for Reactive Attachment Disorder. *APA Monitor*.

De Bellis, M. D., Lefter, L., Trickett, P. K., & Putnam, F. W., Jr. (1994). Urinary Catecholamine Excretion in Sexually Abused Girls. *Journal of the Academy of Child and Adolescent Psychiatry, 33*(3), 320–327.

Delahunta, E. A., & Tulsky, A. A. (1996). Personal Exposure of Faculty and Medical Students to Family Violence. *Journal of the American Medical Association, 275*(24), 1903–1906.

deMause, L. (1998). The History of Child Abuse. *Journal of Psychohistory, 25*, 216–236.

Dubowitz, H., Black, M., Harrington, D., & Verschoore, A. (1993). A Follow-Up Study of Behavior Problems Associated with Child Sexual Abuse. *Child Abuse and Neglect, 17*, 743–754.

Emde, R. N., & Buchsbaum, H. K. (1989). Toward a Psychoanalytic Theory of Affect: II. Emotional Development and Signaling in Infancy. In S. I. Greenspan & G. H. Pollock (Eds.), *The Course of Life: Vol. 1. Infancy*. Madison, CT: International Universities Press.

Erdoes, R., & Ortiz, A. (1984). *American Indian Myths and Legends*. New York: Pantheon Books.

Erikson, E. H. (1950). *Childhood and Society*. New York: Norton.

Erikson, E. H. (1980). *Identity and the Life Cycle*. New York: Norton.

Fair, C. M. (1992). *Cortical Memory Functions*. Boston: Birkhäuser.

Fenton, W. S. (1993). Sexual Abuse and Psychopathology. *Psychiatry, 56,* 205–216.

Fergusson, D. M., & Lynskey, M. T. (1997). Physical Punishment/ Maltreatment during Childhood and Adjustment in Young Adulthood. *Child Abuse and Neglect, 21*(7), 617–630.

Finkelhor, D., Hotaling, G. T., Lewis, I. A., & Smith, C. (1989). Sexual Abuse and Its Relationship to Later Sexual Satisfaction, Marital Status, Religion, and Attitudes. *Journal of Interpersonal Violence, 4*(4), 379–399.

Fivush, R. (1996). Young Children's Event Recall: Are Memories Constructed Through Discourse? In K. Pezdek & W. P. Banks (Eds.), *The Recovered Memory/ False Memory Debate* (pp. 151–168). San Diego: Academic Press.

Fonagy, P., Steele, M., Steele, H., Moran, G. S., & Higgitt, A. C. (1991). The Capacity for Understanding Mental States: The Reflective Self in Parent and Child and Its Significance for Security of Attachment. *Infant Mental Health Journal, 12,* 201–218.

Fraiberg, S., Adelson, E., & Shapiro, V. (1975). Ghosts in the Nursery: A Psychoanalytic Approach to the Problems of Impaired Infant–Mother Relationships. *Journal of the American Academy of Child Psychiatry, 14,* 387–421.

Fraiberg, S. H. (1959). *The Magic Years: Understanding and Handling the Problems of Early Childhood.* New York: Scribner's.

Frankel, F. H. (1993). Adult Reconstruction of the Childhood Events in the Multiple Personality Literature. *American Journal of Psychiatry, 150*(6), 954–957.

Frankel, F. H. (1994). The Concept of Flashbacks in Historical Perspective. *International Journal of Clinical and Experimental Hypnosis, 42*(4), 321–336.

Freud, A. (1963). The Concept of Developmental Lines. *Psychoanalytic Study of the Child, 18,* 245–265.

Freud, A. (1965). Normality and Pathology in Childhood: Assessments of Development. In *The Writings of Anna Freud* (Vol. 6). New York: International Universities Press.

Freud, S. (1953). Three Essays on the Theory of Sexuality. In J. Strachey (Ed. and Trans.), *The Standard Edition of the Complete Psychological Works of Sigmund Freud* (Vol. 7, pp. 125–245). London: Hogarth Press. (Original work published 1905)

Friedrich, W. N. (1993). Sexual Victimization and Sexual Behavior in Children: A Review of Recent Literature. *Child Abuse and Neglect, 17,* 59–66.

Frodi, A. M., Lamb, M. E., Leavitt, L. A., Donovan, W. L., Neff, C., & Sherry, D. (1978). Fathers' and Mothers' Responses to the Faces and Cries of

Normal and Premature Infants. *Developmental Psychology, 14*(5), 490–498.

Gainotti, G., & Caltagirone, C. (Eds.) (1989). *Emotions and the Dual Brain.* Berlin: Springer-Verlag.

Garry, M., & Loftus, E. F. (1994). Pseudomemories Without Hypnosis. *International Journal of Clinical and Experimental Hypnosis, 42*(4), 363–378.

Gazzaniga, M., & LeDoux, J. (1978). *The Integrated Mind.* New York: Plenum Press.

George, C. (1996). A Representational Perspective of Child Abuse and Prevention: Internal Working Models of Attachment and Caregiving. *Child Abuse and Neglect, 20*(5), 411–424.

Gillenwater, J. M., Quan, L., & Feldman, K. W. (1996). Inflicted Submersion in Childhood. *Archives of Pediatric and Adolescent Medicine, 150,* 298–303.

Gillman, R. D. (1992). Rescue Fantasies and the Secret Benefactor. *Psychoanalytic Study of the Child, 47,* 279–298.

Gleaves, D. H. (1996). The Sociocognitive Model of Dissociative Identity Disorder: A Reexamination of the Evidence. *Psychological Bulletin, 120*(1), 42–59.

Goldsmith, S. (1995). Oedipus or Orestes?: Gender Identity Development in Homosexual Men. *Psycholanalytic Inquiry, 15,* 112–124.

Goodman, G. S., Quas, J. A., Batterman-Faunce, J. M., & Riddlesberger, M. M. (1994). Predictors of Accurate and Inaccurate Memories of Traumatic Events Experienced in Childhood. Special Issue: The Recovered Memory/False Memory Debate. *Consciousness and Cognition: An International Journal, 3*(3–4), 269–294.

Gordon, B. N., Schroeder, C. S., Ornstein, P. A., & Baker-Ward, L. E. (1995). Clinical Implications of Research on Memory Development. In T. Ney (Ed.), *True and False Allegations of Child Sexual Abuse* (pp. 99–124). New York: Brunner/Mazel.

Green, A. H. (1995). Comparing Child Victims and Adult Survivors: Clues to the Pathogenesis of Child Sexual Abuse. *Journal of the American Academy of Psychoanalysis, 23*(4): 655–670.

Greenspan, S. I. (1981). *Psychopathology and Adaptation in Infancy and Early Childhood.* New York: International Universities Press.

Grigsby, J., & Schneiders, J. L. (1991). Neuroscience, Modularity and Personality Theory: Conceptual Foundations of a Model of Complex Human Functioning. *Psychiatry, 54,* 21–38.

Grigsby, J., Schneiders, J. L., & Kaye, K. (1991). Reality Testing, the Self and the Brain as Modular Distributed Systems. *Psychiatry, 54,* 39–54.

Halgin, R. P., & Vivona J. M. (1996). Adult Survivors of Childhood Sexual Abuse: Diagnostic and Treatment Challenges. In R. S. Feldman (Ed.), *The Psychology of Adversity* (pp. 147–160). Amherst: University of Massachusetts Press.

Hamilton, E. (1940). *Mythology: Timeless Tales of Gods and Heroes*. New York: New American Library.

Hartman, C. R., & Burgess, A. W. (1993). Information Processing of Trauma. *Child Abuse and Neglect, 17* 47–58.

Heineman, T. V. (1994, April). *How Do You Treat What You Cannot Speak?: The Paradox of Language in the Treatment of Abused Children*. Paper presented at the annual meeting of the American Psychological Association, Washington, DC.

Herman, J. L. (1992). *Trauma and recovery*. New York: Basic Books.

Hewitt, J. W. (1993). Moving from the Language of Action to the Language of Words. In L. B. Boyer & P. Giovacchini (Eds.), *Master Clinicians—On Treating the Regressed Patient* (pp. 259–277). New York: Jason Aronson.

Hewitt, S. K. (1994). Preverbal Sexual Abuse: What Two Children Report in Later Years. *Child Abuse and Neglect, 18*(10): 821–826.

Hicks, R. A., & Gaughan, D. C. (1995). Understanding Fatal Child Abuse. *Child Abuse and Neglect, 19*(7), 855–863.

Horn, M. (1997, July 14). A Dead Child, A Troubling Defense. *U.S. News & World Report*, pp. 24–28.

Howe, M. L., Courage, M. L., & Peterson, C. (1996). How Can I Remember When "I" Wasn't There?: Long-Term Retention of Traumatic Experiences and Emergence of the Cognitive Self. In K. Pezdek & W. P. Banks (Eds.), *The Recovered Memory/ False Memory Debate* (pp. 121–149). San Diego: Academic Press.

Inhelder, B., & Piaget, J. (1958). *The Growth of Logical Thinking from Childhood to Adolescence: An Essay on the Construction of Formal Operational Structures*. New York: Basic Books.

Ions, V. (1983). *Indian Mythology*. New York: Peter Bedrick Books.

Katz, S. M., Schonfeld, D. J., Carter, A. S., Leventhal, J. M., & Cicchetti, D. V. (1995). The Accuracy of Children's Reports with Anatomically Correct Dolls. *Developmental and Behavioral Pediatrics, 16*(2), 71–76.

Kaufman, J., Birmaher, B., Clayton, S., Retan, A., & Wongchaowart, B. (1997). Case Study: Trauma Related Hallucinations. *Journal of the American Academy of Child and Adolescent Psychiatry, 36*, 1602–1605.

Kihlstrom, J. F. (1994). Hypnosis, Delayed Recall, and the Principles of Memory. *International Journal of Clinical and Experimental Hypnosis, 42*(4), 337–345.

Kluft, R. P. (1996). Treating the Traumatic Memories of Patients with Dissociative Identity Disorder. *American Journal of Psychiatry, 153*(7), 103–110.

Krieger, M. J., Rosenfeld, A. A., Gordon, A., & Bennett, M. (1980). Problems in the Psychotherapy of Children with Histories of Incest. *American Journal of Psychotherapy, 34*(1), 81–87.

Krystal, H. (1978). Trauma and Affects. *Psychoanalytic Study of the Child, 33*, 81–116.

Krystal, H. (1979). Alexithymia and Psychotherapy. *American Journal of Psychotherapy, 33*(1), 17–31.

Krystal, H. (1985). Trauma and the Stimulus Barrier. *Psychoanalytic Inquiry, 5*, 131–161.

Krystal, H. (1988). On Some Roots of Creativity. *Psychiatric Clinics of North America, 11*, 475–491.

Krystal, H. (1990). An Information Processing View of Object-Relations. *Psychoanalytic Inquiry, 10*, 221–251.

Krystal, H. (1991). Integration and Self-Healing in Post-Traumatic States: A Ten Year Retrospective. *American Imago, 48*(1), 93–118.

Laub, D., & Auerhahn, N. C. (1993). Knowing and Not Knowing Massive Psychic Trauma: Forms of Traumatic Memory. *International Journal of Psycho-Analysis, 74*, 287–302.

Lawrence, K. J., Cozolino, L., & Foy, D. W. (1995). Psychological Sequelae in Adult Females Reporting Childhood Ritualistic Abuse. *Child Abuse and Neglect, 19*(8) 975–984.

Lieberman, A. F. (1993). *The Emotional Life of the Toddler.* New York: Free Press.

Loewald, H. W. (1979). The Waning of the Oedipus Complex. In *Papers on Psychoanalysis* (pp. 384–404). New Haven: Yale University Press.

Loewald, H. W. (1985). Oedipus Complex and Development of Self. *Psycho-analytic Quarterly, 54*, 435–443.

Loftus, E. F. (1993). The Reality of Repressed Memories. *American Psychologist, 48*(5), 518–537.

Mahler, M. S. (1974). Symbiosis and Individuation: The Psychological Birth of the Human Infant. *Psychoanalytic Study of the Child, 29*, 89–106.

Mapes, B. E. (1995). *Child Eyewitness Testimony in Sexual Abuse Investigations.* Brandon: Clinical Psychology.

McCauley, J., Kern, D. E., Kolodner, K., Dill, L., Schroeder, A. F., Dechant, H. K., Ryden, J., Derogatis, L. R., & Bass, E. B. (1997). Clinical Characteristics of Women with a History of Childhood Abuse: Un-healed Wounds. *Journal of the American Medical Association, 277*(17), 1362–1368.

Meadow, R. (1993a). False Allegations of Abuse and Munchausen Syndrome by Proxy. *Archives of Disease in Childhood, 68*, 444–447.

Meadow, R. (1993b). Non-accidental Salt Poisoning. *Archives of Disease in Childhood, 68*, 448–452.

Mercer, S. O., & Perdue, J. D. (1993). Munchausen Syndrome by Proxy: Social Work's Role. *Social Work, 38*(1), 74–81.

Miller, D. A. F., McCluskey-Fawcett, K., & Irving, L. M. (1993). The

Relationship between Childhood Sexual Abuse and Subsequent Onset of Bulimia Nervosa. *Child Abuse and Neglect, 17,* 305–314.

Mitchell, S. A. (1991). Contemporary Perspectives on Self: Toward an Integration. *Psychoanalytic Dialogues, 1*(2), 121–147.

Moeller, T. P., Bachmann, G. A., & Moeller, J. R. (1993). The Combined Effects of Physical, Sexual, and Emotional Abuse during Childhood: Long-Term Health Consequences for Women. *Child Abuse and Neglect, 17,* 623–640.

Mulhern, S. (1994). Satanism, Ritual Abuse, and Multiple Personality Disorder: A Sociohistorical Perspective. *International Journal of Clinical and Experimental Hypnosis, 42*(4), 265–288.

Myers, J. E. B. (1992). *Legal Issues in Child Abuse and Neglect.* Newbury Park, CA: Sage.

Nash, M. R. (1994). Memory Distortion and Sexual Trauma: The Problem of False Negatives and False Positives. *International Journal of Clinical and Experimental Hypnosis, 42*(4), 346–362.

Newberger, C. M., & Cook, S. J. (1983). Parental Awareness and Child Abuse: A Cognitive-Developmental Analysis of Urban and Rural Samples. *American Journal of Othopsychiatry, 53*(3), 512–524.

Newberger, C. M., & de Vos, E. (1988). Abuse and Victimization: A Life-span Developmental Perspective. *American Journal of Othopsychiatry, 58*(4), 505–511.

Nolte, J. (1989). *The Human Brain: An Introduction to Its Functional Anatomy.* St. Louis, MO: Mosby.

Noshpitz, J., & King, R. (1991). *Pathways of Growth: Essentials of Child Psychiatry: Vol. I. Normal Development.* New York: Wiley.

Novick, J., & Novick, K. (1994). Externalization as a Pathological Form of Relating: The Dynamic Underpinnings of Abuse. In A. Sugarman (Ed.), *Victims of Abuse: The Emotional Impact of Child and Adult Trauma.* Madison, CT: International Universities Press.

Ogden, T. (1997). *Reverie and Interpretation: Sensing Something Human.* Northvale, NJ: Jason Aronson.

Ornitz, E. M. (1991). Developmental Aspects of Neurophysiology. In M. Lewis (Ed.), *Child and Adolescent Psychiatry: A Comprehensive Textbook.* Baltimore: Williams & Wilkins.

Ornitz, E. M., & Pynoos, R. S. (1989). Startle Modulation in Children with Posttraumatic Stress Disorder. *American Journal of Psychiatry, 146*(7), 866–870.

Ornstein, P. A., & Myers, J. T. (1996). Contextual Influences on Children's Remembering. In K. Pezdek & W. P. Banks (Eds.), *The Recovered Memory/ False Memory Debate* (pp. 211–223). San Diego: Academic Press.

O'Shaughnessy, E. (1988). The Invisible Oedipus Complex. In E. B. Spillius (Ed.), *Melanie Klein Today: Vol. 2. Developments in Theory and Practice, Mainly Practice.* (pp. 191–205). London: Routledge.

Pearson, W. S. (1988). The Psychoaggressive Stages of Psychological Development in an Authority-Based Socialization Process. *American Journal of Psychoanalysis, 48*(4), 328–346.

Perry, B. D., Pollard, R. A., Blakley, T. L., & Baker, W. L. (1995). Childhood Trauma, The Neurobiology of Adaptation, and "Use-Dependent" Development of the Brain: How "States" Become "Traits." *Infant Mental Health Journal 15*, 271–291.

Perry, N. W. (1995). Children's Comprehension of Truths, Lies, and False Beliefs. In T. Ney (Ed.), *True and False Allegations of Child Sexual Abuse* (pp. 73–98). New York: Brunner/ Mazel.

Person, E. S., & Klar, H. (1994). Establishing Trauma: The Difficulty Distinguishing between Memories and Fantasies. *Journal of the American Psychoanalytic Association, 42*(4), 1055–1081.

Pezdek, K., & Roe, C. (1996). Memory for Childhood Events: How Suggestible Is It? In K. Pezdek & W. P. Banks (Eds.), *The Recovered Memory/ False Memory Debate* (pp. 197–210). San Diego: Academic Press.

Putnam, F. W. (1988). The Switch Process in Multiple Personality Disorders and Other State-Change Disorders. *Dissociation, 1*(1), 24–32.

Putnam, F. W. (1993). Dissociative Disorders in Children. Behavioral Profiles and Problems. *Child Abuse and Neglect, 17*, 39–45.

Rakic, P. (1991). Development of the Primate Cerebral Cortex. In M. Lewis (Ed.), *Child and Adolescent Psychiatry: A Comprehensive Textbook.* Baltimore: Williams & Wilkins.

Reber, K. (1996). Children at Risk for Reactive Attachment Disorder: Assessment, Diagnosis and Treatment. *Progress: Family Systems Research and Therapy, 5* 83–98.

Rogers, M. L. (1995). Factors Influencing Recall of Childhood Sexual Abuse. *Journal of Traumatic Stress, 8*(4), 691–716.

Ruffman, T., Olson, D. R., Ash, T., & Keenan, T. (1993). The ABC's of Deception: Do Young Children Understand Deception in the Same Way as Adults? *Developmental Psychology, 29*(1), 74–87.

Sarnoff, C. (1976). *Latency.* New York: Jason Aronson.

Sauzier, M. (1989). Disclosure of Child Sexual Abuse: For Better or for Worse. *Psychiatric Clinics of North America, 12*(2), 455–469.

Schaaf, K. K., & McCanne, T. R. (1994). Childhood Abuse, Body Image Disturbance, and Eating Disorders. *Child Abuse and Neglect, 18*(8), 607–615.

Schacter, D. L., Coyle, J. T., Fischbach, G. D., Mesulam, M. M., & Sullivan, L. E. (Eds.). *Memory Distortion: How Minds, Brains, and Societies Reconstruct the Past.* Cambridge, MA: Harvard University Press.

Schaer, I. J. (1994, April). *Action as Metaphor: The Evocative Transference.* Paper presented at the annual meeting of the American Psychological Association, Washington, DC.

Schore, A. (1994). *Affect Regulation and the Origin of the Self: The Neurobiology of Emotional Development*. Hillsdale, NJ: Lawrence Erlbaum.

Schore, A. N. (1997). Interdisciplinary Developmental Research as a Source of Clinical Models. In M. Moskowitz, C. Kaye, & S. Ellman (Eds.), *The Neurobiological and Developmental Basis for Psychotherapeutic Intervention* (pp. 1–72). Northvale, NJ: Jason Aronson.

Seligman, S., & Shanok R. S. (1996). Erikson, Our Contemporary: His Anticipation of an Intersubjective Perspective. *Psychoanalysis and Contemporary Thought, 2*, 339–365.

Settlage, C. F. (1980). The Psychoanalytic Theory and Understanding of Psychic Development during the Second and Third Years of Life. In S. I. Greenspan & G. H. Pollock (Eds.), *The Course of Life: Vol. 1. Infancy and Early Childhood* (pp. 523–539). Washington, DC: U.S. Department of Health and Human Services.

Shengold, L. (1988). Dickens, Little Dorrit, and Soul Murder. *Psychoanalytic Quarterly, 57*, 390–421.

Shengold, L. (1989). *Soul Murder: The Effects of Childhood Abuse and Deprivation*. New Haven: Yale University Press.

Sivan, A. B. (1991). Preschool Child Development: Implications for Investigation of Child Abuse Allegations. *Child Abuse and Neglect, 15*, 485–493.

Solomon, S. (1985). Anatomy and Physiology of the Central Nervous System. In H. I. Kaplan & B. J. Sadock (Eds). *Comprehensive Textbook of Psychiatry*. Baltimore: Williams & Wilkins.

Spence, D. P. (1994). Narrative Truth and Putative Child Abuse. *International Journal of Clinical and Experimental Hypnosis, 42*(4), 289–303.

Stern, D. N. (1985). *The Interpersonal World of the Infant*. New York: Basic Books.

Steward, M. S., Bussey, K., Goodman, G. S., & Saywitz, K. J. (1993). Implications of Developmental Research for Interviewing Children. *Child Abuse and Neglect, 17*, 25–37.

Strichartz, A. F., & Burton, R. V. (1990). Lies and Truth: A Study of the Development of the Concept. *Child Development, 61*, 211–220.

Summit, R. C. (1983). The Child Sexual Abuse Accomodation Syndrome. *Child Abuse and Neglect, 7*, 177–193.

Terr, L. C. (1990). *Too Scared to Cry: Psychic Trauma in Childhood*. Grand Rapids, MI: Harper & Row.

Terr, L. C. (1991). Childhood Traumas: An Outline and Overview. *American Journal of Psychiatry, 148*(1), 10–19.

Terr, L. C. (1996). True memories of childhood trauma: Flaws, absences, and returns. In K. Pezdek & W. P. Banks (Eds.), *The Recovered Memory/ False Memory Debate* (pp. 69–80). San Diego: Academic Press.

Tessler, M., & Nelson, K. (1996). Making Memories: The Influence of Joint Encoding on Later Recall by Young Children. In K. Pezdek & W. P.

Banks (Eds.), *The Recovered Memory/ False Memory Debate* (pp. 101–120). San Diego: Academic Press.

Tobey, A. E., & Goodman, G. S. (1992). Children's Eyewitness Memory: Effects of Participation and Forensic Context. *Child Abuse and Neglect, 16,* 779–796.

Toth, S. L., & Cicchetti, D. (1996). Patterns of Relatedness, Depressive Symptomatology, and Perceived Competence in Maltreated Children. *Journal of Consulting and Clinical Psychology, 64*(1), 32–41.

Toth, S., Cicchetti, D., Macfie, J., & Emde, R. N. (1997). Representations of Self and Other in the Narratives of Neglected, Physically Abused, and Sexually Abused Preschoolers. *Development and Psychopathology, 9,* 781–796.

Tyson, P., & Tyson, R. (1990). *Psychoanalytic Theories of Development: An Integration.* New Haven, CT: Yale University Press.

van der Kolk, B. A., & Fisler, R. E. (1994). Childhood Abuse and Neglect and Loss of Self-Regulation. *Bulletin of the Menninger Clinic, 58*(2), 145–168.

van der Kolk, B. A., Greenberg, M., Boyd, H., & Krystal, J. (1985). Inescapable Shock, Neurotransmitters, and Addiction to Trauma: Toward a Psychobiology of Post Traumatic Stress. *Biological Psychiatry, 20,* 314–325.

van der Kolk, B. A., Perry, J. C., & Herman, J. L. (1991). Childhood Origins of Self-Destructive Behavior. *American Journal of Psychiatry, 148*(12), 1665–1671.

van der Kolk, B. A., & van der Hart, O. (1991). The Intrusive Past: The Flexibility of Memory and the Engraving of Trauma. *American Imago, 48*(4), 425–454.

Watkins, J. G., & Watkins, H. H. (1990). Dissociation and Displacement: Where Goes the "Ouch"? *American Journal of Clinical Hypnosis, 33*(1), 1–19.

Winnicott, D. W. (1958). *Collected Papers.* New York: Basic Books.

Winnicott, D. W. (1971). Transitional Objects and Transitional Phenomena. In *Playing and Reality* (pp 1–25). New York: Basic Books. (Original work published 1953)

Winnicott, D. W. (1994). Hate in the Countertransference. *Journal of Psychotherapy Practice and Research, 3,* 350–356.

Young, J. Z. (1985). What's in a Brain? In C. W. Coen (Ed.), *Functions of the Brain* (pp. 1–10). Oxford: Clarendon Press.

Index